Intersections of Children's Health,
Education, and Welfare

Education Policy

Series Editors

Lance D. Fusarelli, North Carolina State University
Frederick M. Hess, American Enterprise Institute
Martin West, Harvard University

This series addresses a variety of topics in the area of education policy. Volumes are solicited primarily from social scientists with expertise on education, in addition to policymakers or practitioners with hands-on experience in the field. Topics of particular focus include state and national policy, teacher recruitment, retention, and compensation, urban school reform, test-based accountability, choice-based reform, school finance, higher education costs and access, the quality instruction in higher education, leadership and administration in K-12 and higher education, teacher colleges, the role of the courts in education policymaking, and the relationship between education research and practice. The series serves as a venue for presenting stimulating new research findings, serious contributions to ongoing policy debates, and accessible volumes that illuminate important questions or synthesize existing research.

Series Editors

LANCE D. FUSARELLI is a Professor and Director of Graduate Programs in the Department of Leadership, Policy and Adult and Higher Education at North Carolina State University. He is coauthor of *Better Policies, Better Schools* and coeditor of the *Handbook of Education Politics and Policy*.

FREDERICK M. HESS is Resident Scholar and Director of Education Policy Studies at the American Enterprise Institute. An author, teacher, and political scientist, his books include *The Same Thing Over and Over: How School Reformers Get Stuck in Yesterday's Ideas* and *Common Sense School Reform*.

MARTIN WEST is an Assistant Professor of Education in the Graduate School of Education at Harvard University. He is an Executive Editor of *Education Next* and Deputy Director of Harvard's Program on Education Policy and Governance.

Ohio's Education Reform Challenges: Lessons from the Frontlines
Chester E. Finn, Jr. Terry Ryan, and Michael B. Lafferty

Accountability in American Higher Education
Edited by Kevin Carey and Mark Schneider

Freedom and School Choice in American Education
Edited by Greg Forster and C. Bradley Thompson

Gentrification and Schools: The Process of Integration when Whites Reverse Flight (forthcoming)
Jennifer Stillman

Intersections of Children's Health, Education, and Welfare
Bruce S. Cooper and Janet D. Mulvey

Intersections of Children's Health, Education, and Welfare

Bruce S. Cooper and Janet D. Mulvey

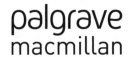

palgrave
macmillan

INTERSECTIONS OF CHILDREN'S HEALTH, EDUCATION, AND WELFARE
Copyright © Bruce S. Cooper and Janet D. Mulvey, 2012.

All rights reserved.

First published in 2012 by
PALGRAVE MACMILLAN®
in the United States—a division of St. Martin's Press LLC,
175 Fifth Avenue, New York, NY 10010.

Where this book is distributed in the UK, Europe and the rest of the world,
this is by Palgrave Macmillan, a division of Macmillan Publishers Limited,
registered in England, company number 785998, of Houndmills,
Basingstoke, Hampshire RG21 6XS.

Palgrave Macmillan is the global academic imprint of the above companies
and has companies and representatives throughout the world.

Palgrave® and Macmillan® are registered trademarks in the United States,
the United Kingdom, Europe and other countries.

ISBN: 978–0–230–34014–5

Library of Congress Cataloging-in-Publication Data

Cooper, Bruce S.
    Intersections of children's health, education, and welfare /
Cooper, Bruce S., Janet Mulvey.
        p. cm.—(Education policy)
        ISBN 978–0–230–34014–5 (hardback)
        1. Children with social disabilities—Education—United States.
2. Educational equalization—United States. 3. Child welfare—
United States. 4. Children—Health and hygiene—United States.
I. Mulvey, Janet D. II. Title.

LC4091.C655 2012
371.93—dc23   2012002816

A catalogue record of the book is available from the British Library.

Design by Newgen Imaging Systems (P) Ltd., Chennai, India.

First edition: September 2012

10 9 8 7 6 5 4 3 2 1

Printed in the United States of America.

Contents

Figures and Tables

Figures

Tables

Foreword

Herbert J. Walberg

In this splendid, scholarly book, Dr. Bruce S. Cooper and Dr. Janet D. Mulvey identify the factors essential to improving the lives of children and adolescents. The authors provide an in-depth look at the tragic, debilitating effects of poverty in America and the accompanying deficits on health and education based on the most important and current research on these three interrelated factors.

They identify important historical perspectives on the factors—health, education, and welfare—and provide examples of effective, successful programs that work to combat their triple scourge. They offer insightful solutions and strong directions for policy makers and decision makers to improve the health, education, and welfare of US children and their families.

The authors identify and examine the mutual causation among the factors and their separate and joint effects on child development and consequences for their adult life. They argue that wise, efficient investments in education improve personal well-being as well as community and national economies. Education accomplishments, for example, insure access to employment, wealth, and better medical care. The effects of poverty, however, include inadequate health care, childhood disease and obesity, poor school attendance, high school dropout rates, underemployment, unemployment, and incarceration.

Although the authors point out evidence on the injurious effects of dropping out of school, they do not argue that higher education is for all. Rather, adopting the perspective of John Dewey, they maintain that effective education integrates subject matter and theory with practical ideas and experiences, providing such examples as (1) learning about politics, democracy, and government by running for political office at school; (2) applying principles of physics and geometry in the context of a school construction and building project; (3) hanging school art projects involving students, art departments, and community professionals in a collaborative mural project; and (4) connecting work and play through sport, teamwork, and competitions such as spelling bees, debate, music, and band.

Drs. Cooper and Mulvey also describe programs that connect education and health-service programs such as the Harlem Success Academy
with records of effectiveness on education, health, and welfare outcomes.
However, the usual programs are disconnected with one another to the
great disadvantage of the economically disadvantaged—and a national
economic loss of an estimated $17 billion annually.

The authors devote a chapter to the influences of family wealth and
income on education, and note the constructive effects of private schools
in diminishing the negative impact of family poverty on children's outcomes. Other positive effects can result from out-of-school enrichment
programs, tutoring services, and summer camps.

Since too few of the programs described are within the reach of many
American needful children and adolescents in poverty, the authors
describe the need for adult education programs concentrated on adult
knowledge and skills in several fields that are most promising for them.
Adult training can result in an increased access to jobs, additional skills
and income in present jobs, and new jobs with better pay and benefits.

Schools can play a vital role in linking services for children, adolescents, and adults. They can serve as community centers and provide
meeting places for service partners involved in health, education, and
welfare support. They can help to foster a sense of belonging, greater
safety, productivity, and self-esteem particularly in neighborhoods where
a dearth of resources and unsafe housing create a climate of distrust, isolation, and stressors associated with poverty. The authors make a case
for full-service community schools for the inner-city and other high-
needs schools and cite examples including Jane Addams's Hull House
in Chicago; Benjamin James High School in East Harlem, NY; and the
Mission School in Boston—all of which had succeeded in breaking the
intergenerational cycle of poverty, ill health, and school failure.

In the concluding chapters, Cooper and Mulvey note the effects of the
education gaps between whites and minorities, and between middle-class
and poor students. They urge a narrowing of these gaps so that more of
American youth can reap the benefits from a college education and gain
better career options, greater monetary benefits, and higher standards
of living. These goals are likely to be more fully realized by employing
the policies, programs, and practices that the authors clearly identify and
describe. For this reason, this impressive book should be highly useful
to those working in the fields of health, education, and welfare, and to
families and children into the twenty-first century.

Part I

Introducing the Problems

This first section explains the thesis of the book: that our children must have good health, and strong education, and be well cared for, if our society is to prosper. It begins, and to some degree, ends, with our children. The "trinity" of this book—health, education, and welfare—is often disconnected in our public policies, and the three fields seem to ignore each other. However, it all must come together with the child.

1

Connecting Health and Education: Improving the Lives of All Children

Children need more than just good schooling: they require safe lives, good health, and sufficient resources to live and grow successfully in their community. This book makes this vital connection, as society must promote a quality education, available and appropriate health services, and financial equity and opportunity for all. Without all these benefits—health, education, and welfare—a child cannot hope to learn, be healthy, and enjoy a good life.

We examine the absence of, or limitations on, children's health services, and then work to relate healthy living to better education, and improved income to well-being. These important connections will mean that children will get the best possible opportunity for education—and thus be focused on learning and growing—and practicing healthy lifestyle habits. Today, New York City public schools reported that 40 percent of school-age children in the city were obese, indicating poor personal habits and lifestyles; a lack of motivation; and a limited opportunity to play athletics, engage socially, and be active in their communities.

The old days of Little League, church dinners, and playing with friends in the neighborhood have passed away, being replaced by kids sitting alone, with bad diets, long hours watching TV and playing on the child's computers and other tech-toys, and poor lifestyles and activity modeling provided by the family.

On top of limited, "virtual" athletics on a computer and a sedentary lifestyle, children today are less likely to have access to regular pediatric services, and to receive quality routine checkups and treatments for various conditions. Emergency rooms may often replace a visit to a neighborhood pediatrician, and are used only when dire, life-threatening medical problems arise.

Therefore, health problems that are routine and straightforward to treat (e.g., asthma, lead poisoning, ear or eye infection, and flu and colds) may go unnoticed. These poor health conditions, besides affecting children's growth and well-being, also often increase absenteeism and even truancy from school.

All of these conditions, educational and health related, are often exacerbated by the poverty of the family and community, and their inability to recognize and get treatment for a range of serious medical problems. These conditions can become "life sentences" that affect children's ability to attend school, graduate, find jobs, and support themselves and their families over a lifetime.

This Book

This book puts the pieces together—intersecting health, education, and welfare—and proposes ways of improving children's health, education, and living conditions, and thus, their contributions to their communities and society. For children who live near or below the poverty line in the United States are more likely to do worse in school, and drop out without completing a high school education.

The effect of persistent poverty and lack of education results in a continuance and perpetuation of low-paying employment or welfare assistance. Lower levels of education have been shown to be indicators of poor health practices, absenteeism in schools, and the inability to procure and sustain employment. This first chapter frames the book, and connects the "triple-condition" of improving health, welfare, and education—to make for a better life.

Connections and Interconnections

As shown in Figure 1.1, we see the three elements of a good life (health, wealth, and education), but we also need to explore and relate these qualities to each other, as the interactions are two-way, meaning, six "connections" can be made.

1--Education Quality

"Good life . . ."

2--Income/Prosperity <--------------- > 3--Good Health & Well-being

Figure 1.1   Connecting the Elements of a Good Life.

1. Connecting Education to Income: Economists (see Levin and McEwan, 2002) have long sought to show that "investing" in children's (people's) minds and education pays big dividends for the individual with better jobs and higher income (measured often as increase in their "lifetime earning streams").

Likewise, Theodore W. Schultz, a University of Chicago economist and winner of a Nobel Prize for Economic Sciences, found that investing in education increased the US gross domestic product (GDP) by enabling citizens to get better jobs, earn higher incomes, and thus buy and use/consume more goods and services (homes, vacations, and cars), improving the economy. As Schultz (1992 wrote in his autobiography:

> The adverse economic events following the First World War turned me toward economics. In the Dakotas, where I was born (April 30, 1902), I learned during my youth how hard it was for farm families to stay solvent. Farm product prices fell abruptly by more than half. Banks went bankrupt and many farmers suffered foreclosures. Was politics or economics to blame? I opted for economics. (p. 705)

Schultz (1961) went on to show that investing public resources in education paid off for all three levels: (1) personal growth and income of individuals, (2) benefits to the community having well-educated citizens, and (3) dividends to the society with higher incomes, more productivity, and stronger consumption—the qualities of a better GDP (and Gross National Product [GNP]), that is, the sum of the value of all production and consumption, public and private.

In addition, Eliot A. Jamison, Dean T. Jamison, and Eric A. Hanushek (2007) found internationally that "the economic impact of improved cognitive ability at a country-wide level complemented and extended similar findings at the individual level" (p. 3), thus investment in education improves growth nationally, and provides benefits for each person.

Further, they assert that

> ISATs [International Student Assessment Tests] in mathematics appear to be measuring an element of human capital that is important to growth in income per capita and that is not captured by quantity (years) of schooling on its own. This effect is quantitatively important: depending on the specific assumptions, a one standard deviation increase in test scores is associated with an increase in annual growth in income per capita of 0.5–0.9 percent (with our preferred model at the low end of the range).

2. Relating Family Income to Education: The other relationship, income to education, is easier to see. Just visit a fancy suburb, or classy neighborhood in the city; note the clean, well-run schools, with parents visiting and students prospering. Economists, too, study how both high- and middle-income families have children more likely to attend a good school, graduate high school, get into college and professional school, and go on to a career of choice (Murnane et al., 2000).

Conversely, poor neighborhoods, with unemployed and underemployed families, may often have less productive schools, which are less likely to graduate students, who will be struggling to go to college and/ or get good jobs. Perhaps, the strongest study of this situation is Henry Levin's research on boys of color, who have lower incomes and get less-effective education. They then go on to be sicker, poorer, more likely to be on welfare, and to get into trouble with the police. Levin et al. (2007) explained the relationships as follows:

> When we add up the three public benefits of education [better health, less crime and incarceration, and better income]…the value of just the public benefits embodied in tax revenues and reduction in the cost of public health and crime amounts to almost $257,000 per new high school graduate. (p. 706)

Jonathan Kozol blew the lid off the differences in income and school quality, finding in his classic book, *Savage Inequalities* (1991) that richer New York City suburban schools spent more than double the poorer inner-city district amounts. As Kozol explained: "The story was the same throughout the country: per-capita spending for poor students and students of color in urban areas was a fraction of that in richer, whiter suburbs just miles away" (p. 112). Thus, more money means better schools, putting poor children of color at a real disadvantage, as those districts with the highest proportion of black students often receive less local and state funding.

So, more money—higher income—means better schools. So, why did this happen? According to Michael Rebell, former executive director of the Campaign for Fiscal Equity, lawsuits have produced some changes. "New Jersey, for instance, began channeling funds to its poorest districts after a court challenge [*Abbott v. Burke,* 100 N.J. 269, July 1985]; as of 2000, the state government provided roughly three times as much per capita funding to the poorest quarter of districts as it did to the richest quarter (Rebell, 2009, p. 32). And students from well-off homes, living in more prosperous communities, besides getting a better local education, are much more likely to graduate high school and attend and graduate college.

3. Higher Income, Better Health Services, and Mortality: The next relationship is virtually of life and death, as families with lower incomes are less likely to get good medical services, be healthy, and live longer. Meredith Minkler et al. (2006) at University of California-Berkeley found that a poor family of four (earning below $17,761 income per year) was *six times* more likely to suffer ill health and disabilities than richer families that make seven-times that amount or more. We all know that the poor live and work in less-healthy settings, and are thus more likely to be ill—even extending into the lower-middle class.

As Minkler et al. (2007) explained: "The fact that there's a significant difference between people at 600 percent and 700 percent above the poverty level was a striking finding of this study" (p. 696). So more wealth means better health, longer life, and the opportunities to prosper as a family. Income insures that the individual gets good medical care as a child, growing into adulthood, and throughout the rest of life. Illness, as we know, is a complex condition, that may require hospitalization, operations, treatments, and careful drug consumption.

The United States has been among the slowest of modern nations to offer full socialized medicine, unless one is terribly poor and on welfare; and even then, getting treatments may require much time on line, waiting to be "called into" the doctor of nurses' offices, and then lines to get free drugs and services. Having a regular, private doctor (general practitioner) and a slew of specialists for every different medical condition is a great expense that most lower-middle-class and poor families and individuals cannot afford. Thus, the costs of good care are high, as a regular checkup can cost $500, a treatment can cost thousands, and an operation with following can be over $25,000 per condition.

Being well-off and well employed often guarantees better and more medical care and hospitalization insurance, and extra resources for medicines and treatment in and out of hospital. In addition, medical problems can grow, get more complex, and require a number of drugs and treatments if they are not caught and treated earlier and well.

4. Better Health, Better Life Opportunities: Turn the equation around: the healthier people are, the more likely they are to sustain work, make progress, have time and energy to be active in their communities, and care for their children and families. Sick people cannot work, are hardly able to bring in a regular income, and struggle to make economic progress. As a promotion for the State of Colorado, where health is a way of life, explained: "Healthier people are more energetic. Healthier students learn better."

Hence, healthier families may be happier. "And a healthier workforce is more productive and reduces employer health-care costs." In some cases, we hear the opposite argument, sadly, that sick people are *good*—even profitable:

A car crash is good for the economy—by traditional measurements. Ambulance companies make money from accidents; emergency medical technicians pick up overtime. So do healthcare workers, body-and-fender shops, car dealerships and the car companies, insurance adjusters, physical therapists, and psychotherapists. All these are counted by traditional economic measures, and in those measures probably far outweigh the lost capital represented by any un-depreciated value of the destroyed cars—and may even outweigh the costs of the lost work hours and lowered lifetime productivity of the injured, and the hiring and training costs to replace the dead. (Hawken, 1993, p. 94)

Hence, what is not measured—or what is not considered measurable in traditional economics—is the human suffering and despair. These feelings are dismissed as an "intangibles." Paul Hawken (1993), in *The Ecology of Commerce*, says:

To create an enduring society, we will need a system of commerce and production where each and every act is inherently sustainable and restorative. We must design a system...where doing good is as like falling off a log, where the natural, everyday acts of work and life accumulate into a better world as a matter of course, not a matter of conscious altruism. (p. 22)

Hawken (1993) mentions an interesting case of how to sustain society, its people and actually improve productivity and the quality of life. They are Menominee Indians of Michigan who have a private forest of 243,000 acres right next to the Nicolet National Forest. The national forest is over twice as large, but the Menominee consistently get far more board feet of usable lumber out of their forest. Are they clearing-while-cutting?

No. They cut carefully, selectively. Every seven to ten years they survey the forest, and at each survey over the last 40 years the forest has more trees, more lumber, increased bio-mass. They have been doing this for more than 135 years. The asset on which they make their living is said to be a beautiful place: a recent study declare that "aesthetically [it] has no equal among managed forests in the Lake States region." (Hawkins, 1993, p. 14)

The magnitude and power of such research has grown tremendously in recent years. Two things have pushed it into the spotlight. First, the stunning rise in health-care costs throughout the 1980s and into the early 1990s brought business into a desperate search for ways of cutting health-care spending.

Second, business made health care its partner in this search by forcing health care to take on risk for covered lives. For the first time, as health care becomes at risk (or "at profit," we might say) for the health of populations, the financial life and death of institutions depended on increasing the health of populations through nonmedical means. The magnitude of the stakes involved are illustrated by studies undertaken in conjunction with major insurance companies, which show $6 saved for every $1 spent on nonmedical methods of reducing heart disease.

5. Better Education, Better Health: Next, we can connect being well schooled with being healthier. Much of health and well-being can relate to how well read, learned, and intellectual one is. Exercising, eating well, and knowing what are best lifestyle decisions and practices can all be related to having the ability to read, think, and reason.

Better-educated people are healthier—because they keep up with the latest trends in diet, exercise, and medical treatment—and know how and when to visit their doctor(s). And when something medically does go wrong, they can get the best treatments and make the right choices. As one account explains: "After a year of constant jabbering about medical care, last month's heated debate and President Obama's signature just days ago, this celebrating of National Public Health Week might seem anti-climatic. It's not."

Rather, this weak call—with its emphasis on health literacy and preventive care—seems a perfect segue into a decade of progress in medicine. "An educated public is essential to improving individual health and wellness," says Georges C. Benjamin, MD, executive director of the American Public Health Association. "Today's technological era allows patients to be better informed."

6. Better Health, Better Education: The United States lags behind most industrialized nations in math and science education. The usual grumble on this—that we're losing our competitive edge in industry and technology—is a matter of business, a concern leading corporations such as Westinghouse and Intel to sponsor science competitions and Congress to enact bills such as the "America COMPETES Act" of 2007.

But in the matter of health, whether it is private or public, so little is said about the boon of education mixed with enhanced, public access to medical information and technology. Furthermore, being educated can also prevent the rise in expensive medical treatments, as the *American Journal of Public Health* highlights:

> *Primary disease prevention is not only good for our health, but also our budgets;*
> *Connections exist between neighborhoods and the risk of chronic disease onset in later life; and*
> *Urban areas with smaller food markets may be bad for our waistline.*
> (Dwyer, 1986, pp. 1287–1288)

Thus, primary disease prevention is not only good for our health, but also for our budgets. In a new study from the *American Journal of Public*

Health, researchers found that primary disease prevention would lead to huge potential national and state medical-care savings.

Bringing It Together

Thus, this book has an important mission and message: to show how ridiculous it is to talk about better education without relating schooling to decent parent income and better heath. The "trinity" of health, education, and income/welfare is so essential together, interacting, that to discuss any one or two of these alone, is foolish. One cannot disconnect the universal public goal of *education* from *resources* (private and community wealth and funds) and *health*—as the three interact, and helping or hindering each other, truly making sense together.

This book will treat each dimension—educating; financing; and sustaining families, children, and individuals—together, and at the same time will show just how they interact and improve each other. Healthy people can work, learn, and improve. In addition, educated people know how to make money, educate themselves and their offspring, and receive good health care—to everyone's benefit.

References

Dwyer, J. (1986). Reducing the great American waistline. *American Journal of Public Health. 76*(11, 1287–1288.

Hawken, P. (1993). *The ecology of commerce: A declaration of sustainability.* New York: HarperCollins Publishers.

Jamison, E. A., Jamison, D. T., & Hanushek, E. A. (2007). The effects of education quality on income growth and mortality decline. *Economics of Education Review. 26*, 772–789.

Kozol, J. (1991). *Savage inequalities: Children in America's schools.* New York: Crown Publishers.

Levin, H. M., Belfield, C., Muennig, P., & Rouse, C. (2007). The public returns on public educational investments in African-American males. *Economics of Education Review, 26*(1), 700–709.

Levin, H. M., & McEwan, P. J. (Eds.), (2002). *Cost-effectiveness and educational policy.* Lachmont, NY: Eye on Education.

Minkler, M., Vasquez, B. V., Warner, J., Stuessey, H., & Facente, S. (2007, August 17). Health and wealth: together. *The New England Journal of Medicine, 355*(2), 695–703.

———. (2006). Sowing the seeds of sustainable change: A community-university research and action partnership in Indiana and its aftermath. *Health Promotion International, 21*(4), 293–300.

Murnane, R. R., Willett, J. B., Duhaldeborde, Y., & Tyler, J. H. (2000, Fall). How important are the cognitive skills of teenagers in predicting subsequent earnings? *Journal of Policy Analysis and Management, 19*(4), 547–568.

Rebell, M. A. (2009). *Courts and kids: Pursuing education equity through the state courts.* Chicago, IL: University of Chicago Press.

Schultz, T. W. (1961). Investment in human capital. *The American Economics Review, 51*(1), 1–17.

———. (1992). *Nobel lectures, economics 1969–1980.* Assar Lindbeck (Ed.). Singapore: World Scientific Publishing Co.

2

Serving School Dropouts: Who Are They, What Can Be Done?

Introduction

The United States continues to develop as a society that requires ongoing learning skills to give meaning and solve problems in an ever-evolving technological world. The competitiveness in the international marketplace has become intense, increasing the pressure to produce a citizenry able to produce new knowledge on a daily basis. Improving education for future generations is the most important investment in human capital for our future prosperity—locally, nationally, and internationally.

The difference in achievement of students in more- or less-affluent social classes should be a concern for overall national health and prosperity. Lack of investment in education for students in poor neighborhoods has caused a loss of revenue and productivity in the United States. Too many students, with poor educational backgrounds, dropout of school, costing the nation billions each year in lost work, higher welfare payments, and reduced production.

The dropout rate from the nation's high schools is thus a concern for the economy, productivity, and competitiveness in the international marketplace. As the economy declines, increasing the national debt, and devaluing the US Treasury Bonds, we need to examine one causal factor that drains instead of contributes to the financial health of the nation. Dropouts from high school are at an all-time high. According to the US Department of Education, National Center for Education Statistics, 1.2 million students fail to graduate on time with a regular diploma each year. Of extra concern is the demographic concentration of minority and low-income groups whose children never get a high school diploma. With numbers of high school dropouts on public assistance increasing and productiveness declining, we need to examine national and local policy on unrealistic educational standards requiring the same academic programs for all.

This chapter will study the dropout rate statistics, provide research data on schools and programs, and make recommendations in program electives, schools, and funding. Locating the lowest-performing high schools, we will follow a backward timeline to seek causes of poor results, based on students and family's health, income, and economic status. For now, another adolescent student drops out of school every nine seconds in America. What do we know and what can we do? Can we overcome political bias, examine the problem realistically, and adopt fair measures to serve all youth in America?

History

Prior to the opening of public high schools in the late 1800s, boys from the wealthy classes were educated in private academies and/or by tutors preparing them for college. Middle-class boys were offered secondary education, once the merchant, craftsman businesses, and commerce became more prevalent in society.

Early high schools did not admit girls or minorities. Not until the late 1800s were girls accepted into "Normal Schools" to receive their training to become elementary school teachers. According to Fenske (1997), in 1900, some 6,000 high schools graduated only 6 percent of American 17-year-olds.

Then, secondary education in the United States became more popular in the early 1900s, supported by American labor unions; and according to Welter (1962), public education "pursued the fundamental strategy of substituting education for other techniques of social action in attempts to cope with social problems" (p. 189). Funding high schools through taxes had its supporters and detractors, creating arguments from those who had the resources to pay for private education. The issue was resolved in 1874, when the Michigan Supreme Court (the *Kalamazoo* Case) ruled in favor of tax support for public high schools. The court decision allowed families, unable to pay for private academies, to send their children for secondary school education training at no personal expense (Raubinger and Piper, 1969).

Curriculum for the Masses

Attendance in the secondary school increased dramatically: by 1930, some 30 percent of adolescents in the United States were attending high school. The growth in attendance divided the students between those who would or would not attend college. This division thus demanded a curriculum that prepared all students to be productive for themselves and their communities, whether they went on to higher education or not. Progressive educators believed that curricula choices should be differentiated and include "practical courses" and vocational training to prepare students for employment and later life.

A report by the National Education Association, *Cardinal Principles of Education* (1918), recommended "that secondary education focus on health, the command of fundamental principles, worthy home membership, vocation, citizenship, worthy use of leisure time, and ethical character" (p. 11). High school education became a universal, comprehensive reality encompassing the ever-diverse needs among students. The NEA committee argued that the schools should meet the needs of "a widely diverse student population…needs could be met though varied curriculum options relevant to the needs of current students" (p. 12).

Graduation Rates in Decline

Statistically, today, three out of ten students in the United Sates will dropout of high school. According to the Editorials Projects in the Education Research Center, high school completion fell by .04 percent in 2007 and now stands at 68.8 percent in 2011. These findings mark the second consecutive year of decline and fall in areas that are most vulnerable in terms of resources and income. Swanson (2010) reports that where we see the most decline and disengagement is in poor communities. He states that, "the effects of the graduation crisis fell disproportionately on the nations most vulnerable youths and communities…majority of non graduates are members of historically disadvantaged minorities and underserved groups" (n.p.). Students in these communities attend large underresourced urban high schools with less experienced teachers, large classes and undifferentiated curriculum.

Historically the population attending high schools increased exponentially from the 1920s to the 1940s. High school graduation was established as goal for employment and possible postsecondary education or training. The completion peak was recorded in 1969 with 77 percent of youth earning diplomas. Currently according to Swanson (n.d.), "The next three decades were marked by a retreat from those historical highs; the graduation rate eroded incrementally…including a large drop in the early 1960s…the graduation rate now stands at about the same level as it did in the early 1960s" (n.p.).

Cost to the Nation

The cost to society for uneducated youth is high in areas of poor health, unemployment, and in too any cases, incarceration. Marc H. Morial, a former New Orleans mayor, now the president of The National Urban League, describes the dropout problem succinctly in an article by Sam Dillon in the *New York Times* (2009), "The dropout rate is driving the nation's increasing prison population, and its drag on America's competitiveness . . . every American pays a cost when a young person leaves school without a diploma."

Just as the graduation rates have declined over the last three decades, so has earning power followed suit. Reports indicate that those youth who have left school without a diploma have a jobless rate as high as 55 percent. And those working earn less than half of their graduating peers. The Center for Labor Market Studies (2004) reveals that between 1997 and 2001, of all dropouts, 25 percent were unemployed for more than a year, compared to 11 percent of those with diplomas or General Education Development (GED) certificates (Khatiwade, Sum, and McLaughlin, 2004). The increase in unemployment rises to more than 50 percent of young African American males in 2003.

A study done by the Center for Labor Market Studies at Northwestern University, using data from census forms and government statistics, found that one of every ten high school dropouts is either in jail or in a youth detention center. The cost to society for each incarcerated teenager is approximately $292,000 annually. According to Sum (2011), "It [incarceration] is one of the country's costliest problems."

Also, importantly, the preponderance of arrests, convictions, and imprisonments occur among young male minorities who have grown up in poor neighborhoods with few resources and little societal support, educationally or economically. Also, female dropouts were nine times more likely to become single mothers without means of support, thus having to rely on public assistance, food stamps, charity, and welfare. Generational perpetuation of uneducated people, who are dependent solely on public assistance, must be addressed and remediated.

The costs to local, state, and national treasuries are affected by the expenses for public assistance, food stamps, emergency health care, and criminal incarceration, all connected with the lack of educational attainment. The following are some of the costs to the American public due high school dropouts:

- Earning power comparison: In 2003, for example, income was $21,477 for high school dropouts; $32,266 for high school graduates; $43,462 for those with an Associates degree; and $63,084 for college graduations with a bachelor's degree.

- Health-care cost comparisons: $41.8 billion a year in health-care costs are incurred by high school dropouts.
- Public welfare costs: $10.8 billion are spent annually for food stamps, housing assistance, and temporary assistance for needy families.
- Crime costs: $1.4 billion cost is associated with court and incarceration.
- Lost resources over a lifetime: $260 billion are in lost wages, lost taxes, and lost productivity over a lifetime.

These statistics must be announced, heard, and heeded, according to Seastrom (2005) and others, because "every nine seconds in America, a student becomes a dropout!" (p. 12).

In addition, in an article in London's *The Daily Telegraph*, on September 2, 2011, Rowley reported that 370,000 families in several generations have never even held a job. According to the article, England has seen an increase of families where one in fifty children has never witnessed a family member work or earn a living. Thus, "in total, about 1.8 million children live in households where their parents do not work" (p. 1).

The employment opportunities, lifetime earnings, and social status are all dependent on the quality and completion of an education. Educational quality not only affects an individuals earning power, but also is an indicator or prediction of whether people are "to be unemployed, living in poverty, receiving public relief, in prison on death row, unhealthy, or single parents" (US Department of Labor, Bureau of Labor Statistics, 2008).

Most of the welfare subsidy goes to single mothers who have become welfare dependent, and findings show that welfare dependence is deleterious for children's development. Rector (1999) found that "current research indicates that both welfare dependence and single parenthood...impedes children's ability to become successful members of society and...prolonged welfare dependence reduced children's IQs" (p. 1).

The vicious cycle of poverty—depression, anger, abuse, neglect, addiction, anxiety, and a sense of worthlessness—are perhaps the primary contributors to the dropout crisis. Curriculum demanding academic preparation for college for all is not only unreachable and ridiculous, but also sets unrealistic and impossible goals for many students, rich or poor.

Curriculum and Standards

Controversy and Contention

How do the current curriculum requirements affect the graduation rate, for students who reside in lower-class communities and attend large urban or poor rural schools?

The economy was and is a major influence on education in the United States and abroad. As jobs demanded more education and training, politicians and educators encouraged more schooling for its youth. During the 1940s and 1950s, a differentiated curriculum remained in place, allowing students to select courses that would align with their interests and employment aspirations. In 1944, the Educational Policies Commission issued a report encouraging a practical curriculum that would produce graduates ready for the workplace, or a more academic curriculum for those aspiring for a postsecondary education.

The economy and its practical implications continued to influence curriculum and programs until 1983, when *A Nation at Risk* was published. The report warned of decline in the international market place and lack of economic competitiveness. The recommendations made by the National Commission of Excellence in Education were to raise standards, and develop a rigorous curriculum for all students whether college bound or not. The report blamed tracking for academic "mediocrity" and proposed more rigorous curricula for all.

The report initiated a challenge to face our issues of deficiency and to become a competitive force in international educational ranking. Changes were made to educational standards and measurement of achievement. The biggest change came in 2001, when the *No Child Left Behind* legislation made testing and accountability the mantra for public education. As a result, according to the US Department of Education in *A Nation Accountable* (2008), "We are now able to see how well each of the approximately 96,000 public schools in our country is performing" (p. 8).

The outcomes of the current academic focus and test-ready preparation have not changed our status on international rankings. We are, at best, remaining stagnant and worse falling behind some third world countries. Where the United States was once, according to the Organisation for Economic Co-operation and Development (OECD) (2007), "the leader in high school completion rates, but among 25–34 year olds, it has now fallen to 10th place" (p. 7). And on international tests, the United States is on a slippery slope downward. Perhaps, we should become alarmed when according to Loveless (2001), "with performance like this, it is no wonder that most foreign children studying in the United States find our schools easier than the ones they left back home" (p. 12).

Current programs in public schools, elementary through high school, have become test-driven "factories." Curriculum is propelled by state mandated and standardized tests. The arts and extracurricular activities have either been curtailed or eliminated to provide more time and resources for test preparation and academic intervention services. Students who fail or score "below proficient" are mandated to take remedial classes. Some schools require before- or after-school remediation, making it difficult for students to become engaged in clubs or extracurricular interests.

High schools have instituted double periods for academic subjects to assure preparation and the passing of standardized tests given for school and district rating. Gone are the electives of yesteryear and vocational programs for talented students whose learning styles and/or motivation go beyond the current basic mandated academic subjects.

High-stakes tests, having often replaced electives and vocational programs, are first experienced as young as in kindergarten for placement and remediation focus. The tests designed to assess readiness, teacher effectiveness, and school proficiency have failed the most important elements in school: the students. In a report by the National Board, evidence suggests that high-stakes assessments are linked to increased noncompletion or dropouts.

Indicators link together high-stakes tests, low-socioeconomic status. and dropout rates. In states that educated the largest populations of low-income students, the National Board found the highest dropout rates and maximum use of the high-stake tests for decisions concerning promotion or graduation. A study done through National Longitudinal Surveys, National Center for Education Statistics (2000), examined and found that "students who had to pass one or more minimum competency tests in eighth grade were more likely to drop out of school by tenth grade" (p. 2).

All evidence indicates that high-stake tests are not improving our educational system or helping us to be competitive in international standing. Falling further behind, we need to adjust our paradigm for excellence to stop the downward spiral.

Changing Paradigms for Reform

Key indicators show that using high-stake tests for promotion or graduation is leaving many young people behind. The development of curriculum and programs based on the contents on those tests is superficial, analogous to Piaget's description of the "banking system"—teaching by depositing information for regurgitation. Dropouts from low-socioeconomic areas are just one indicator of our failing system. Another sign of the "banking system" of teaching and learning is the lack of preparation for the more rigorous challenges in college. Teaching without engagement in higher level, critical thinking, exploration, and discovery and instead focusing on test preparation inhibits the skills necessary for understanding and applying knowledge on a higher level.

Sharon Otterman (*New York Times,* February 11, 2011) reported that only 23 percent of New York City's high school graduates are ready for college; and of those who attend, many are in need of remedial classes. In response, the state is looking to raise standards, toughen tests, and hold schools and administrators accountable. This plan sounds like more of the same. If conditions for teaching and learning or the paradigm for reform do not change, improving results will be negligible, if at all, and such continuous practices might exacerbate the dropout problem for students already struggling.

What Can We Do? How Can We Begin?
Where Do We Start?

Policy makers, state and local officials must recognize the intersection of education with the economy, social stability, and democratic ideals, if we are to continue to participate and lead in the international marketplace.

High school reform cannot continue on its current path of using inapplicable tests as indictors of success. Expectations that all students should pursue academic content geared to higher education are also unrealistic. Continuing with current reform experiments can lead to even wider achievement gaps, more dropouts and worse economic repercussions.

The largest percentage of dropouts comes from low-socioeconomic groups and minority populations. The lost revenue in monetary value and human capital due to dropping out of school is staggering and unnecessary. We can no longer ignore the statistics that link poverty, health, and the dropout population.

To begin to address the issues connected to perpetuation of poverty and lack of employment skills, we need to start at the beginning. For policy makers and those in power to make changes, leaders must accept responsibility for economic commitment to health, childcare, and early childhood education. Parents on public assistance should be expected to pursue training or education to become more self-sustaining. Housing should be safe and free from toxic elements that affect health and cognitive functioning of the young child or adult.

Examining the most successful education system in the world (in Finland) can enlighten and compare principles that create success among 99 percent of youth versus the increasing issues of failure (United States). As Mulvey (2011) explains, "It is time to examine our schooling practices, curricula standards, core curriculum and assessment models for success and failure" (p. 1). What are some comparable accommodations to take to change the outcomes for all students, in particular, those who suffer inequities due to socioeconomic circumstances?

1) Health care for all should be a right not a privilege. All the citizens in Finland have access to health care and are treated with preventive services avoiding the "too late" emergency visits that cause death or disability.
2) Preschool available for all children is highly affordable and subsidized according to the family's ability to pay, and curriculum for the youngest child is centered on the national core curriculum and involves play and discovery instead of content-driven material.
3) All schools are equally funded, class sizes are the same, and the quality of teacher is constant across all socioeconomic levels.
4) Teachers are respected, paid equally and fairly, and follow a standard core curriculum that is adaptable and applicable.
5) Students are separated in their last three years in high school, according to their interests and skill levels. Approximately 53 percent of students study more academic courses and the remaining enter vocational school.

The result in another country: Finland has a dropout rate of 4 percent, as students are prepared to earn a living based on their skills and interests; they are independent and contribute to the wealth and prosperity for themselves and their country.

America's mantra, "College for Everyone," has been disastrous for students, teachers, schools, and districts in the nation, leaving us far behind internationally in literacy, math, and science. Schools pressured to reach the mandated goals have proven catastrophic, leading to practices deleterious to all involved, especially the students.

Attention to the pressure for passing these state and national tests was brought to light on July 7, 2011, in an article that made national news. Jeneba Ghatt (2011) of the *Washington Times* wrote, "Revealing that nearly 200 Atlanta school administrators, principals and teachers changes children's text scores...an investigation by the state of Georgia calls into question whether the controversial 'No Child Left Behind Act' may be contributing to cheating at school systems nationwide" (p. 1).

Policy and Politics for Better Schools, Successful Students

How do we change the mindset of policy makers so they can understand the underlying causes for lack of achievement, removing blame from the poor and initiating policies for success?

Can we initiate success by ignoring the health needs of uninsured children? Mandate goals without initial preparation for learning? Unequally fund wealthy and poor schools? And when do we see future consequences of current policies?

On August 26, 2011, just prior to the opening of the public schools in New York City, the mayor Michael Bloomberg announced staff layoffs, hitting the poorest city's school districts most in need, "sparing the affluent ones." Juan Gonzales (2011) in the *New York Daily News* explained that the Department of Education's layoffs hit poorest areas hardest. Blaming city councils in the poorest areas for the layoffs, the mayor and chancellor distanced themselves from the most needy children, causing even more hardship in educating the city's poor.

The mayor's action is consistent with many policy makers who cater to their political base and neglect those with little influence. Their actions are direct contributions to school failure and dropout numbers. Result? Exacerbation and perpetuation of generational school failure and dependence on government-subsidized programs.

Real Reform Preventing Dropouts

Children's preschool experience is crucial for success. C. T. Ramey and S. L. Ramey (2004) report, "Children's experiences prior to kindergarten entry are correlated with degree of cognitive development and school readiness... children from economically poor and uneducated families are at elevated risks for lack of school readiness due to lack of knowledge and skill" (p. 471).

Research conducted with randomized controlled trials emphasizing experiences necessary for learning found that preschool for high-risk children was efficacious in improving later academic success. As Shonkoff and Phillips (2000) confirm, "children who do not have early transitions to school—are those most likely to become inattentive, disruptive, or withdrawn... later are the students most likely to drop out" (p. 3).

From Neurons to Neighborhoods

Providing universal daycare and preschools for children living in high-poverty areas is a first preventive step in the dropout rate. Language development, cognitive stimulation, and social experience provide an incentive to learn more and succeed. All learning is based on language, understanding, and use. Hart and Risely (1995) studied the interrelationship of language use and interactions between families and their children in upper, middle, and poor classes for a two-and-half-year span.

Their findings demonstrate the difference in language acquisition and readiness for formal schooling. Data reveal a wide gap, such as knowledge of just 500 words of three year olds living in impoverished conditions compared to 1,000 words for children in more-affluent settings. The differences persisted, were predictive of children's proficiency, and evident on third-grade standardized assessments in reading, language, and comprehension.

Early childhood programs should best be conducted with certified teachers, and standardized in terms of core curriculum goals for cognitive and social development. C. T. Ramey and S. L. Ramey (2004) assert, "the well being and school readiness of our nation's children needs to be a major priority so that all children receive the essential transactions and learning opportunities vital for their brain development" (p. 478). Assessments should be used as tools to develop individual profiles on the strengths and the weaknesses in readiness for learning.

Funding for resources—class size; safe, pleasant physical structures; and teacher quality—needs equity disbursement, ensuring that all students in school have similar opportunities and experiences. Strong leadership is needed to develop and convince all policy makers on the need for comprehensive educational initiatives serving differentiated skill and interest levels.

Vocational schooling and apprenticeship during the last three years of high school—preparing noncollege bound students for careers in areas of choice—will avoid failure and motivate students to complete school and graduate with skills. Vocational schooling for the twenty-first century involves high technology in all industries and should be an integral part of all vocational training. A 2001 report on *NPR*, "A high school dropout's midlife hardships," (Sanchez, 2001) touted the usefulness of and employment opportunities for students with technologic skill. The report on July 28, 2011, outlined the need for software developers, programmers, and other tech personnel for companies in their competition to amass and execute new materials.

High schools should remain up-to-date in opportunities for their students' future employment, and design and implement programs to meet the growing twenty-first-century needs. The opportunities must reflect all service needs, professional, business, labor, and technology to support an economy ever and evermore diverse.

Conclusion

The number of the nation's high school dropouts is a major concern for the health of our country. The drain on the economy (e.g., GDP) from nonproductivity, incarceration, petty crime, poor health, and welfare subsidies continues to increase; and in the current financial downturn more Americans find themselves unemployed, causing an even greater strain on our economic system.

The uneducated find themselves with fewer opportunities to work or earn salaries above the poverty level. Perpetuation of dependence on the social service sector has become a generational expectation. The intention of welfare programs is temporary relief until more gainful employment can be found and financial independence established. As generations of families become dependent on a system providing sustenance, no positive role models emerge for children in those families to instill the value of work, independence, and opportunity for personal growth. Anne Hill and June O'Neill (1990) describe the effects of welfare dependence on children's lowered IQ.

Schools in high-poverty areas have been unsuccessful in providing the basic motivation and skills that make learning attractive and meaningful. High-stake tests fail to accommodate the needs of poor children's lack of language and experience in primary grades. Labeling as early as kindergarten—and failing by third grade—are nonincentives for learning, which continue through the mandatory ages for schooling. Most children, who have been unsuccessful in their early years and have often been retained one or more times, drop out as soon as possible.

Schools that are academic only—seeking to make all students college ready and higher education bound as the answer for viability in employment and fiscal independence—must be reexamined. Expecting all students to have similar cognitive structure is unrealistic and leaves too many children behind and unproductive.

Universal preschool for all children, especially those in poor and impoverished areas, is critical for the development of language and experiential readiness for formal education. Electives in vocational and technical training in our high schools will provide a rich alternative to purely academic pursuits.

Policy makers on the local and national levels must reexamine their priorities, in school reform. Evidence suggests that more tests, less program diversity, unequal funding, and less resources, all have failed to benefit the students, the economy, or the nation. John Dewey (2009) succinctly explained the role of education as preparing for the ongoing and inescapable process of change: To prosper as a country and society, education for all is our best hope.

References

Center for Labor Market Studies (2004). *Dire straits in the nation's labor market: The outlook for the summer 2010 teen job market and the case for a comprehensive youth jobs creation strategy.* Northeastern University, Flint Michigan April 2010. Prepared for C. S. Mott Foundation 2010.

Dewey, J. (2009). *Democracy and education: An introduction to the philosophy of education.* New York: Macmillan.

Dillon, S. (2009). *Study finds high rate of imprisonment among dropouts.* Retrieved from www.nytimes.com/2009/10/09/education/09/dropout.html.

Fenske, Neil, R. (1997). *A history of American public high schools 1890–1990: Through the eyes of principals.* Lewiston, NY: Edwin Mellon Press.

Ghatt, J. (2011, July 7). Atlanta's cheating ways: School officials changed test scores. *The Washington Times.*

Gonzales, J. (2011). Department of education layoffs hit poorest areas hardest. Retrieved from http://articles.nydailynews.com/2011–08–26/local29947262.

Hart, B., & Risely, T. R. (1995). *Meaningful differences in the everyday experience of young American children.* New York: Brooke Publishing.

Hill, M. A., & O'Neill, J. O. (1990, March). *Underclass behaviors in the United States: Measurement and analysis of determinants.* New York: City University of New York, Baruch College.

Kalamazoo Case 1874 (2001). In National Center for Education Statistics.

Khatiwade, I., Sum, A. & McLaughlin, J. (2004). *The labor force behaviors, employment and earnings experiences, and labor market problems of the disabled working-age population in Massachusetts, New England, and the u.s. In 2003 and 2004.* Boston: Northeastern University: Center for Labor Market Studies Publications.

Loveless, T. (2001). How well are American students learning? *The 2001 Brown Center Report on American education.* Washington, DC: The Brookings Institution.

Mulvey, J. D. (2011). Applying Finland's, paradigm to NYC kids. *The school administrator, 68*(11), np.

National Center for Education Statistics (2000). *Dropout rates in the United States.* Washington, DC: Author.

National Commission of Excellence in Education (1983). *A Nation at Risk.* Washington, DC: Author

National Education Association (1918). *Cardinal principles of education.* Washington, .

Otterman, S. (2011, February 7). Most New York students are not college-ready. *The New York Times.*

Organization for Economic Co-operation and Development. *Education at a glance 2007: OECD indicators.* Paris, France: Organization for Economic Co-operation and Development.

Parker, W.C. ed. (1996.) *Educating the democratic mind.* Albany, NY: SUNY Press.

Ramey, C. T., & Ramey, S. L. (2004). Can early learning and school readiness as early intervention make a difference? *Merrill-Palmer Quarterly, 50*(4), 471–491.

Raubinger, R., & Piper, W. (1969). *The development of secondary education.* New York: Macmillan.

Rector, R. (1999, May 11). The effects of welfare reform: Testimony on welfare and welfare spending. *Report of the Center for Data Analysis, The Heritage Foundation.*

Rowley, E. (2011, September 2). Global slowdown hitting manufacturing. *The Daily Telegraph*, City Desk, p. 1.

Sanchez, C. (2011, July 28). A high school dropout's midlife hardships. *NPR.*

Seastrom, M. (2005). *The averaged freshman graduation rate for public high schools from the common core of data.* Washington, DC: U.S. Department of Education, National Center for Educational Statistics.

Shonkoff, J., & Phillips, D. A. (2000). *From Neurons to neighborhoods: The science of early childhood development.* Washington, DC: National Academy Press.

Sum, A. (2011). *National youth employment center.* Retrieved from www.nyec. org/page1D.

Swanson, C. B. (2010). U.S. graduation rate continues to decline. *Education Week.* Retrieved from http://www.edweek.org/articles/2010/06/10/34.

US Department of Education (2008). *A Nation Accountable: Twenty-five years after A Nation at Risk.* Washington, DC: Author, Retrieved from www.ed.gov/ rschstat/research/pubs/accountable.

Welter, R. (1962). Hidden curriculum and the nature of conflict. In Parker, W. C. (1996). *Educating the democratic mind.* Albany, NY: State University of New York Press, pp. 173–200.

Part II

Understanding the Disconnections

This second section tries to explain why the three needs (health, education, and welfare) are treated as separate field, concerns, and disciplines, whereas they are tightly connected theoretically and empirically. Economists such as Henry Levin and Theodore Schultz have shown that education costs money, but pays back in a larger GDP and less crime, better health, and of course, improved income. Why the disconnect? And how to reconnect?

3

Higher Education Is Not for Everyone: What about Vocational-Technical Education and Useful Skills?

Introduction

Remember this great joke?

A prominent neurosurgeon is having plumbing problems in her home, and calls a prominent plumber in the neighborhood. Arriving with tools and replacement pipes, the plumber removes the metal sink pipes that are leaking and replaces them with new modern plastic pipes in about 3 hours. He presents the doctor with a bill for $2,300 for the work.

The doctor examines the bill, is truly amazed, and says to the plumber: "Looking at your charges, I think you make more per hour than I do!" The plumber thought for a moment, and said, "Yes, I believe you're right. I do make more money now as a plumber than I did when I was a surgeon."

Joke or not, no matter how electronic, postmodern, and hi-tech our society becomes, we shall always need craftspeople and skilled technicians to do heating, electrical and plumbing work, building construction and repairing, car repairs, and equipment use, as well as instillation and maintenance. And as our society becomes more and more highly technical and electronic, the training of men and women who can work with their hands will become ever more important.

So, how can adult learning and training centers, located in community centers or schools, provide technical and skill-center education, preparing adults for vocational and technical work, which will always be important in construction, maintenance, and new high-technology work?

We see solutions in several areas:

1) Reintroduce vocation-technical education in high schools and community colleges, to give formal, practical training in key areas;
2) Bring education and voc-tech companies together, to place and train students in real-life settings with benefits for both schools and industry;
3) Relate and use practical exercises in teaching all school subjects, to reinforce learning and retention; and
4) Use creative play and hands-on applications in teaching and learning in kindergarten through high school and beyond.

1. Reintroduce Voc-Tech Education

Students once took voc/tech-education at school, as skill areas were learned and practiced along with their basic cognitive-academic subjects. Why not offer these skills to all students, as electives (such as athletics and gym), as useful activities that do not necessarily have to become a career—but that build useful skills: for example, changing a light bulb, fixing a lawn-mower, building a dog house or bird bath (Nadel, 2002). As one argument goes, technical colleges and institutes teach these skills, so why not make them part of the regular secondary school program?

> As the labor market becomes more specialized and economies demand higher levels of skill, governments and businesses are increasingly investing in the future of vocational education through publicly funded training organizations and subsidized apprenticeship or traineeship initiatives for businesses. At the post-secondary level vocational education is typically provided by an institute of technology, or by a local community college. (Wikipedia http://en.wikipedia.org/wiki/Vocational)

Joe L. Kincheloe (1995) wrote a useful book, *Toil and Trouble: Good Work, Smart Workers, and the Integration of Academic and Vocational Education,* that makes a key point: Students can certainly learn much from practical skills, that can reinforce their knowledge of math and science, and life. And as a summary of the book, Kincheloe explains, "The need to reform schools and integrate vocational and academic education is examined in the context of the political dynamics that connect schools and the economic system" (p. 232).

Kincheloe further argues "that integrating academic and vocational education is a better way of educating students and alerting them to the complexities of the world and the nature of the physical, social, political, and economic reality confronting them" (p. 1).

2. Bring Education Agencies and Technical Firms Together

A second step in vocational education and its connection to academic achievement would be to create national and regional partnerships, between business and public agencies (such as sanitation, public maintenance, city sewer works, and electrical services) and K-12 and higher education centers, to determine what we need in the next generation of technicians and designers, and how best to train and support these critical technical people.

This melding of voc-tech and academic learning would likewise benefit private enterprise, public services, and education at all levels, since these levels and agencies cannot survive without each other. Public service providers need a stream of qualified and highly trained technicians to assure that communities have the necessary services to run safely and efficiently.

Lien, Hung, and McLean (2007), in their article in the *Human Resource Development Quarterly,* found that "organizational learning" (OL) and "organizational development" (OD) are closely related, so that not only are students learning in schools, but also as adults, they continue to study and develop in their jobs, which in turn helps them to improve the performance (and profitability) of companies and other organizations. The authors explain:

> Contributions of organizational learning to organizational performance: First, the extent and capacity of learning, according to respondents, should be driven by top management to organizational performance. Second, the content of learning is influenced by the organizational culture. Third, there was a general observation that organizational learning as an OD intervention promotes sharing and learning of information and experiences from one employee to another in an open and adaptive manner. Such sharing is perceived to influence organizational performance in a positive way. (p. 221)

Thus, firms and schools are somewhat alike. For their members (workers and students respectively) learn best by doing, trying, testing, and working together, as OL relates to OP. And both relate to personal learning (PL). As one manager of a business explained:

> How do we know whether our organization reaches its goals? We have a scorecard to balance employees' performance. For example, everybody in our company should have an ICP [individual competency profile]. We

compare it to his or her position profile, and, if there is a gap, then we provide training or other techniques to help him or her improve...Everybody has his or her own balanced scorecard, and the company has its business-balanced scorecard. If we follow the strategy and deploy it to every level, performance should be OK. (Lien, Hung, and McLean, 2007, p. 222)

Thus, companies, as well as schools, can tie good results (outputs) to the education (training) of the participants (the inputs). Thus, everyone in education, government agencies, and industry needs to keep tabs on the training that members receive and the "balanced scorecard" that relates learning to outcomes. Schools are a business, like industry, and learning is vital to both.

3. Tie Curriculum Theory with Practice

Educators once understood the value of connecting practical, hands-on learning and knowledge to theories and abstract ideas. In fact, "pragmatist" philosopher John Dewey (1859–1953) argued that learning cannot truly occur unless students are taught how to be "problem-solvers"—figuring out how to be problem-solvers—thus helping students learn how to think and act, rather than simply learning rote lessons about large amounts of information.

In fact, Dewey believed that schools should focus on *judgment* rather than *knowledge* so that school children become adults who can "pass judgments pertinently and discriminatingly on the problems of human living" (Campbell, 1995, pp. 215–216).

Dewey also wanted schools to help students learn to live and work cooperatively with others. In *School and Society* (1899), he wrote, "In a complex society, the ability to understand and sympathize with the operations and lot of others is a condition of common purpose which only education can procure" (p. 32). Working cooperatively assumes that schools are focused on common problems, doing joint projects, and demanding that schools work together on real practical matters.

Dewey (1899) summarized his beliefs when he wrote: "Thus, I have attempted to indicate how the school may by connected with life so that the experience gained by the child in a familiar, commonplace way is carried over and made use of there, and what the child learns in schools is carried back and applied in everyday life, making the school an organic whole, instead of a composite of isolated parts" (p. 80). In addition, the results of Dewey's philosophy meant that

Dewey's progressive ideas in the educational philosophical debate entropied. His notion of learning as an activity that promoted autonomous, rugged thinkers seemed in conflict with the other progressive view of harmonious relationships with progress, science and industrialism in an American economy—especially an economy that had the possibilities of dominating the world. Practical education, focused on work place realities, grew nationally, appealing to the industrialists, immigrants, legislators and many other segments of American society. The changes taking place in American society seemed linked to scientific method and industrialization, therefore justified their adoption. By default, practical education became what the culture perceived as worthwhile and proper for the majority of the learners. "The principal object...should be to secure the maximum prosperity for the employer, coupled with the maximum prosperity for each employee." (Wikipedia http://en.wikipedia.org/wiki/John_Dewey)

Schools, then, need to do more than teach subject matter and theories; somehow, education needs to integrate practical ideas and experiences, to test and expand upon the ideas and theories learned in classes, such as math, science, language arts, and history. How can these thoughts and ideas be made practical, and applied and used in everyday life? Vocational and technical education is a good starting point, as students see what works, and how, as part of the concepts of the field. Dewey's notion of education as an "organic whole" benefits everyone. Learning what works, how and why, can expand and reinforce the concepts behind the ideas.

Example 1: Learning about Politics. Running for political office in one's school can teach a student much about how democracy and government work, paralleling the importance of history and social studies in the education of all people. What better ways to understand one's own position, ideology, and sense of power than to read a school's constitution; to define the power and role of student government; to form political coalitions and "parties" based on ideas, gender, ethnicity, and beliefs; and to determine what skills and trades the district is teaching? The power of the vote is more than a principle; it's an operational process in electing and supporting colleagues for office—and helping to govern and improve the school.

Example 2: Constructing and Building. What if a school decided to build a high-tech learning center, where students could plan construction projects, organize their materials and equipment, and apply theories of geometry, physics, and then use them in real conditions? Not only would they see how these theories "come together" in real work and projects, but students and teachers would also begin to see the limits of their work. All these skills could be used in real life, as students moved into the work force as skilled technicians and even innovative inventors.

Example 3: Hanging School Art. Rather than living in schools with long blank walls in the corridors, why not have the art departments plan a theme for each wall, and have students design and execute a Major Mural Project. When Brooklyn Technical High School was constructed to "put workers to work" in the Great Depression in 1935 in New York City, the purpose was to put designers, construction workers, and artists to collaborate in building a public building. In this case, they built a large public technical high school for 4,500 students—to absorb the influx of students to the city—and to create a center for technical and academic learning.

On the top floors, large studios were constructed with sand on the floor, so that students could learn the skills of welding, soldering, and pouring hot metals into casts. On the main floors, large murals were painted as part of the Work Progress Administration (WPA), around themes of history, progress, and mechanical development, which a century later still attract visitors and give the high-tech school an historical feeling.

4. Connect Work and Play

Finally, many schools—and parents—know the value of sports to the growth, skills, fair play, and well-being of children. It's about more than just winning (or losing). It's about teamwork, trusting your colleagues, and seeking a common goal: to win! Spelling bees, debate societies, and even music competitions by orchestra, band, or chorus, all teach students about seeing the world as cooperative and team-oriented, since few jobs in life are working alone and lonely.

Recent research at two universities shows that students learn more and better when they can "act out" their lessons. As one Voc-Tech center explained:

> Vocational schools, colleges and universities, and other specialized trade and technical schools, offer students an exceptional opportunity to advance your education, skills, and overall marketability in today's competitive job market. Whether it's for a career change or simply to expand your knowledge with some additional educational courses, these technical and vocational schools provide a convenient, cost-effective means to obtain specific degrees and certifications. (Vocational and Technical Education Center)

A series of experiments by researchers at Arizona State University in Tempe and at the University of Wisconsin-Madison suggest that students can understand and infer more by physically acting out texts—either in real life or virtually—than by reading alone.

In the most recent of the experiments published in the June issue of the journal *Scientific Studies of Reading*, researchers found that elementary mathematics students who acted out the text in word problems were more accurate and less distracted than those who didn't.

A more-recent math study followed the same format with 97 third- and fourth-graders using math story problems instead of simple algorithms and were thus more engaged and had better understanding of the mathematical concepts. Researchers found that students who acted out the story—and then learned to visualize it mentally—were significantly more likely than the control groups to answer the problems correctly. To a great extent, the active students were 35 percent less likely to be distracted by irrelevant numbers or other information than students who did not act out the text. "Forcing the students to think through the story helped them weed out what information related to the math question," Mr. Glenberg said (Sparks, 2011, p. 22).

Clark Aldrich (2005) explains the value of practical and technical training, and practice in learning and recalling information and skills, through the use of hi-tech approaches and practices as explained in a book:

> Designed for learning professionals and drawing on both game creators and instructional designers, *Learning by Doing* explains how to select, research, build, sell, deploy, and measure the right type of educational simulation for the right situation. It covers simple approaches that use basic or no technology through projects on the scale of computer games and flight simulators. The approach models content as well, written accessibly with humor, precision, interactivity, and lots of pictures. Many will also find it a useful tool to improve communication between themselves and their customers, employees, sponsors, and colleagues. (p. 111)

This approach has many uses and means of learning that bring together concepts, drills, practices, and skill building through practice. As this Aldrich (2005) method explains:

> When it comes to education and training, computer games change everything. Generations of game creators have raised the bar on engagement, and opened the door to new types of material that can be formally learned. At the same time, leading academic, corporate, and military instructors have developed new types of interactive content. Most have worked dramatically better than the traditional alternatives, if only in specific situations. This method covers simple approaches that use basic or no technology through projects on the scale of computer games and flight simulators. (p.112)

The process uses content as well written processing, accessing them with humor, precision, interactivity, and lots of pictures—often through the use of "games for learning."

Vocational Training and Work

We see the value of work, craftsmanship, and cooperation, as keys to improved skills and attitudes that schools need to master. And technical education doesn't end with high school, or technical college. As fields develop, and hardware and software become more advanced, technical training must move innovatively forward. And education never ends. A case in point, made by Motoko Rich (2011), illustrates the need to change and upgrade even the most basic technological skills:

> Mark McSweeney, a 34-year-old former welder, started out trying to improve his skills to find work in a new sector. Halfway through his studies, he lost his job. After two years, he obtained an associate's degree in applied science in the Metals Engineering Technology program at Forsyth Technical Community College in Winston-Salem, N.C., where about three-quarters of the students are people who had been working before returning to college. After Mr. McSweeney completed his degree, he landed a job inspecting electronic parts. (p. 41)

This connections between basic technical and scientific education, mainly in middle and high school, and more advanced technical training in college, are now being well-recognized, as these two levels (tech-science) work together during high school and beyond. Since learning is continuous, education can and should be ongoing. The false breach between high school and college should be bridged to benefit students and their technology growth.

An advertisement in a local Ohio newspaper spells out the options and opportunities created by seeing technical education as a lifelong process:

> **Announcement:** Current high school students can attend the local community college as part of the Post Secondary Enrollment Options (PSEO) program offered in Ohio and Option B qualifies the students to earn college credits that also fulfill their high-school graduation requirements simultaneously. The best part is…all of the courses and the textbooks are FREE…as long as the student meets the required minimum for a passing grade.
>
> Post Secondary Enrollment Options is a cost effective program that more students should apply for and benefit from while in high school. Unfortunately many parents and their students are not aware that this program exists and is available. Guidance Counselors need to be informed of and recommend programs that motivate and benefit students who are prepared for higher learning. (PSEO, University of Minnesota)

Getting Away

We need to move away from overreliance and overuse of standardized tests as measures of growth and achievement; instead we should make greater use of education research and practice. For we see the overuse of passive preparation methods to meet academic standards and achievement, while learners need to have an active, hands-on, concrete, applied, and practical approach to learning, which also improves instruction and testing outcomes.

A market exists for schools that prepare students for careers in technical fields. A group called "the Association of Career and Technical Education" (ACTE) exemplifies the opportunity that this preparation and training presents. As the description of the role of ACTE states:

> Guiding principles of this organization include lifelong learning, competitiveness, and continual improvement of curriculum design in career and technical education...The professional development offers help to new professionals, including teacher tips for vocational teachers and a webcast series designed to show the latest in career and technical education...
>
> The strength of the Association for Career and Technical Education (ACTE) is reflected in its diverse membership composed of more than 27,000 career and technical educators, administrators, researchers, guidance counselors, and others who are involved in planning and conducting career and technical education programs at the secondary, postsecondary and adult levels. (www.acteonline.org/about.aspx)

We, as a society and as educators, need to understand and respect the growing need for skilled workers, service providers, and practical experts. Not everyone is liberal arts and/or pure sciences oriented. Instead, students can chose a range of career paths and practice, once they have mastered basic reading, math, and social skills, in fields that interest and motivate them: education must give them esteem, self-worth, and abilities to earning a living—while they can also help society. These craftspeople are real contributors to society, the economy, and their community!

Examples: Middle Country School District, NY, had a high-end architectural, carpentry, electrical, and plumbing program in the high school. Each year, students explore and follow architectural designs, build a house frame, install electrical, plumbing lines, and then auction off the house for funding of the next project. Also, programs such as Habitat for Humanity help to build partnerships between the public schools, construction and supply companies, and students working in apprenticeship efforts to learn—during their twelfth grade or beyond.

And the homes that they construct can be given to needy families, using a lottery if too many need them. President Jimmy Carter was a great supporter of Habitat for Humanity, and helped hundreds of families to obtain a home, while teaching community cooperation and home-building skills. What could be better for all concerned?

And voc-tech careers can start at any time. As one group explains, individuals can make the ten steps to a new career and new work at any time.

These steps may include the following:

1. Decide If You Need a Career Change

Before you begin thinking about making a career change you have to decide whether you actually need one. You may just need to find a new job, not an easy task, but certainly simpler than an entire career makeover.

2. Assess Yourself

If you decide a career change is in order, you will need to evaluate your values, skills, personality, and interests using self-assessment tools, often called career tests. Self-assessment tools are used to generate a list of occupations that are deemed appropriate based on your answers to series of questions. Some people choose to have career counselors or other career development professionals administer them, but many opt to use free career tests that are available on the Web.

3. Make a List of Occupations to Explore

Look over the lists of occupations generated through your use of the self-assessment tools. They are probably rather lengthy. You want to come up with a much shorter list, consisting of between five and ten occupations.

4. Explore the Occupations on Your List

For each occupation on your list, you will want to look at the job description, educational and other requirements, job outlook, advancement opportunities, and earnings.

5. Continue Narrowing Down Your List

Pare down your list of possible occupations based on what you learned from your research. For example, you may not be willing to put the time and energy into preparing for an occupation for which an advanced degree is required, or you may consider the earnings for a particular occupation inadequate.

6. Conduct Informational Interviews

At this point you should only have a few occupations left on your list. You now need to gather more in-depth information. Your best sources of this information are people who have firsthand knowledge of the occupations in which you are interested. Identify who they are and conduct informational interviews with them.

7. Set Your Goals

By now you should have decided on one occupation you want to pursue. It's time to put a plan in place so you can eventually find a job in that field, but first you will need to set some goals.

8. Write a Career Action Plan

Now that you have set your goals, you will need to decide how to reach them. A career action plan will help guide you as you pursue your long and short-term goals.

9. Train for Your New Career

Changing your career may mean you have to undergo some training. That could take the form of earning a degree, doing an internship or taking courses to learn some new skills.

10. Say Goodbye to Your Current Career

Your decision to change careers may have been inspired by a job loss. In that case you don't have to worry about leaving your job. However, if you are currently employed, you will have to quit your job and deal with some issues related to that (McKay, 2011).

Career programs, make-up and beautician programs, and other vocational preparation once were common; but in the rush for national standards, we have moved to instructing in basic subjects and ignoring practical applications. And in the process, we're sacrificing students' potential and ignoring the everyday needs of society.

References

Association of Career and Technical Education (ACTE), *Career-Tech Vision*, 2012. Retrieved from https://www.acteonline.org/

Aldrich, C. (2005). *Learning by doing: A comprehensive guide to simulations, computer games, and pedagogy in e-learning and other educational experiences.* San Francisco, CA: Pfeiffer.

Campbell, J. (1995). *Understanding John Dewey: Nature and cooperative intelligence.* Peru, IL: Open Court Press.

Dewey, J. (1899). *The school and society.* Chicago: University of Chicago Press. Retrieved from http://en.wikipedia.org/wiki/John_Dewey.

Kincheloe, J. L. (1995). *Toil and trouble: Good work, smart workers, and the integration of academic and vocational education.* New York: Peter Lang.

Lien, B. Y. H., Hung, R. Y., & McLean, G. N. (2007). Organizational learning as an organization development intervention in six high-technology firms in

Taiwan: An exploratory case study. *Human Resources Development Quarterly, 18*(2), 211–228.

McKay, D. R. (2011). How to Make a Successful Career Change. The 10 steps you need to take when you make a career change. Retrieved from http://career-planning.about.com/od/careerchoicechan/tp/career_change.htm.

Nadel, J. (2002). Imitation and imitation recognition: Functional use in preverbal infants and nonverbal children with autism. In A. N. Meltzoff and W. Prinz (Eds.), *The imitative mind: Development, evolution and brain bases* (pp. 63–73). Cambridge: Cambridge University Press.

Post Secondary Education Options (PSEO). Retrieved from http://education.state.mn.us/MDE/StuSuc/CollReadi/PSEO/index.html.

Rich, M. (2011, July 11). Community college as a bridge to new skills. *COMMUNITY COLLEGES—Economix—New York Times,* December 9, 2010, (p. 41).

Sparks, M. (2011, July 13). "Acting Out" text found to promote pupils' learning. *Education Week, 30*(36), 18.

Vocational and Technical Education Center. Retrieved from http://www.vocational-technical-schools.com.

Wikipedia. http://en.wikipedia.org/wiki/Vocational.

4

Connecting and Comparing Education with Health Services

Two of the purposes of major social services in the United States—regardless of family income—is to provide education for children of all abilities and needs, and quality health services for Americans of all ages, regardless of job or income. The availability and quality of both of these programs, however, are often related to the user's job, income, home location, and wealth, although education and health-care services operate very differently in our mildly socialistic—strongly capitalist—country.

Education is compulsory, universal, and free, and perceived as a primary societal way of increasing students' opportunities, participation in society, and later personal income. Health care, in contrast, is associated with work, income, age, and need, and is neither a required public program, nor a universal government service such as compulsory public education. While every state has a constitutional requirement for the provision of a free, local education, health care is neither required nor universal.

While formal K-12 education involves over 55 million children daily, aged 5 to 19, and about 4 million adults (of whom 3.2 million are teachers, and others are administrators, and education specialists), health services treat a smaller number of patients daily, but cost much more annually. From the analysis of cost changes between 2008 and 2009 by "National Health Expenditures" (NHE), we see that

- NHE grew 4.0 percent to $2.5 trillion in 2009, or $8,086 per person, and accounted for 17.6 percent of GDP.
- Medicare spending grew 7.9 percent to $502.3 billion in 2009, or 20 percent of total NHE.

- Medicaid spending grew 9.0 percent to $373.9 billion in 2009, or 15 percent of total NHE.
- Private health insurance spending grew 1.3 percent to $801.2 billion in 2009, or 32 percent of total NHE.
- Out-of-pocket spending grew 0.4 percent to $299.3 billion in 2009, or 12 percent of total NHE.
- Hospital expenditures grew 5.1 percent in 2009, slower than the 5.2 percent in 2008.
- Physician and clinical services expenditures grew 4.0 percent in 2009, slower than the 5.2 percent in 2008.
- Prescription drug spending increased 5.3 percent in 2009, faster than the 3.1 percent in 2008.
- The federal government's share of health-care spending increased just over 3 percentage points in 2009 to 27 percent, while the shares of spending by households (28 percent), private businesses (21 percent) and state and local government (16 percent) fell by about 1 percentage point each. (Department of Health and Human Services, 2009)

Comparing expenses between health care and schooling, while few children are engaged daily in medical services and treatments (thank goodness!), the total national costs of public education in 2009 was $591 billion, while health in 2010 ran $.8 trillion at the federal level. When we look at the sources of public school funding in 2008–2009, we see that the state contributes the majority overall, local districts come second, and the federal share is the smallest. The breakdown is as follows:

Public Education Spending 2008–2009

State sources:	46.7 percent
Local sources:	43.8 percent
Federal sources:	9.5 percent.
Total	$590.9 billion

At the state and local levels in 2010, spending on health services is $526.3 billion, while education was costing $846.2 billion at the state-local level. Thus, total health-care costs are $1.1 trillion in 2010, while education ran $0.9 trillion (US Government Spending.com). Teachers are perhaps the largest public sector employee group, numbering about 3.2 million in the 50 states and the District of Columbia—not counting the additional 365,000 private school teachers.

Interestingly, while education spending is focused on the younger members of society, "per person personal health care spending for the 65 and older population was $14,797 in 2004, 5.6 times higher than spend-ing per child ($2,650) and 3.3 times spending per working-age person ($4,511)" (National Health Expenditures Data www.cms. gov/Resarch-Statistics- Data). We know, however, that ignoring the young and treating the more obvious elderly with illnesses, makes sense in the short run, but none over the years.

Connecting and Comparing Health and Educational Services

The connections among health, education, and ultimate welfare are being recognized, and data are now being regularly gathered and analyzed. For example, the Federal Interagency Forum on Child and Family Statistics published *America's Children: Key National Indicators of Well-Being* (2011) "as a compendium of data on both the promise and the challenges now confronting our Nation's young people" (p. 1).

The forum explains that "this year's report continues to present key indi-cators in seven domains: (1) Family and social environment, (2) economic circumstance, (3) health care, (4) physical environment, and (5) safety behavior, (6) education and (7) health." When these data are put together, the forum is able to connect the services to the child and to society.

Comparing the support of medical and education services, we see that 90 percent of the US children attend public schools at little or no personal cost, and the rest go to private schools or are homeschooled, while 59.3 percent of citizens in the United States go to private medical services often through their employers under private insurance programs such as Blue Cross & Blue Shield and CIGNA. Thus, "an estimated 3.8 million workers are enrolled in consumer-drive plans about equally divided between high deductible plans and plans with a health reimbursement arrangement" (Kaiser Family Foundation, 2007).

This chapter connects and compares these two vital human services—showing the evolution of the two efforts, and their importance in pro-ducing and maintaining a healthy, happy, well-educated, and prosperous nation. We also examine what's being done to reach that goal where these services are not available to everyone equally and adequately. And we learn much from this comparison about how nations work, from the democratic-localist tradition such as the US "village school" movement, to the capitalist free market approach that underlies the delivery of medi-cal and health services.

Recall the sweetly smiling actor Robert Young, seated behind his desk in his clinic, as the general practitioner Marcus Welby, MD, offering kind and caring treatment in a country (1970s) where one anonymous reactor wrote: "The show is about doctor Marcus Welby, a general practitioner and Steven Kiley, Welby's young assistant. The two try to treat people as individuals in an age of specialized medicine and uncaring doctors."

What the commentator forgot to mention was that poor folks have little or no medical care, since they often cannot afford Dr. Marcus's loving services unless he extend it to them out of a sense of charity. For, healthcare coverage in 2007 for the average family was $12,106, while "workers on average now pay $3,281 out of their paychecks to cover their share of the cost of a family policy" (Kaiser Family Foundation, 2007, p. 1).

Thus, while education is there for everyone, though of varying levels of quality, health care is far from available and universal. In fact, health services are becoming more expensive, and fewer families can afford any coverage. In 2007–2008, for example, the percentage of families with no insurance increased by 5 percent. So between 2001 and 2008, "premiums for health care increased 78%, while wages for workers have gone up only 17% and inflation has gone up 19%" (Kaiser Family Foundation, 2007, p. 5).

We know that although Medicaid, for example, is provided to families living at or below the assigned poverty level, real access to health care is difficult to access, particularly for families in rural areas. Since these families are poor, and often lack transportation, they cannot easily access services in regional medical centers and hospitals, where they should be receiving preventative care.

Thus, many do not actually gain access to medical services until an emergency problem occurs. Statistically, younger children with chronic illnesses (60 percent) die within 24 hours when they finally are admitted to a regional hospital. Without preventative and responsive medical care, children suffer from cognitive losses and abilities required for learning in schools. Poor nutrition, poor living conditions, neglect, and no medical services are stressors that can cause less learning and the lowering of IQ, when tested.

In essence, education was always a free-socialized (government-run and government-funded) program (e.g., the original public "village school" supported by local property tax income), required by state compulsory education attendance laws—at either a public or private school (see *Pierce v. Society of Sister,* 1925)—while health care was a pay-as-you-go service that could be costly to the patients and families. The employed, better-off families often had private coverage under programs such as Blue Shield/Blue Cross while poorer or unemployed families got little or no medical help, unless crises emerged and they stood in line (or lay on gurneys) at a hospital emergency room, or qualified by age and/or poverty for Medicare and Medicaid.

Hadley (2003), in *Sicker and Poorer: The Consequences of Being Uninsured,* connects poverty and medical care (and insurance).

These two programs are living examples of how a democratic, free enterprise society can operate an enormous socialistic, government-owned-and-run education system (including about 58 million adults and children who attend daily), and a smaller, more expensive, mixed economic health-care system with insurance as private, often given as a "benefit" in a job. But those who are poor or unemployed may often have no insurance and must seek Medicare for acute illness. Preventative care is less available, excepting basic tests and some vaccinations for flu, small pox, and other illnesses.

How They Connect

If we are to relate health, education, and welfare, comparing education services with medical care is enlightening. We know that socioeconomic status, earned in large part by success in one's job and profession, is a critical determinant of the health care one gets, and is often obtained through education attainment and quality (see Levine, 1998). Thus, "household income" is *both* an indicator of achievement and standing, and the basis for determining access to good health care, and whether one can get a good, if not the best, education for children. Thus, one key attribute of social class is "income," the others are individual and household, as mother and father may both be employed:

Income is one of a set of family attributes most commonly used to determine people's class status. Yet, income alone may not always accurately reflect a household's position within society or the economy. Unlike individual personal income, *household* income does not reflect occupational achievement as much as it measures the number of income earners.

Sociologist Dennis Gilbert (1997) acknowledges "that a working class household with two income earners may out-earn a single-income upper middle class household, as the number of income earners has evolved into one of the most important variables in determining household income" (p. 22).

For example, according to the US Department of Labor, two registered nurses could quite easily command a household income of $126,000 annually, while the median income for a lawyer was $94,930. Furthermore, household income fails to recognize household size. For example, a single attorney, earning $95,000, may have a higher standard of living than a family of four with an income of $120,000. However, household income is still an often-used class indicator, as household members share the same economic fate and class position (Gilbert, 1997, pp. 32–33).

Fussel (1997) concludes, "educational attainment is one of the most prominent determinants of class status. As educational attainment represents expertise, which is a necessary component of the capitalistic market system, its ownership may be seen as the ownership of one of the factors of production" (p. 14). In other words, persons with advanced degrees already own one of the essential buttresses of the economy: they have expertise. Those with higher educational attainment tend to be positioned in occupations with greater autonomy, influence over the organizational process, and better financial compensation.

While economic compensation is merely the result of scarcity, educational attainment may be related to that very economic principle as well. The obtaining of a graduate degree represents the acquisition of expertise, a variable of production, which in itself may be scarce; thus leading to better financial compensation for the owner.

As explained above, the upper-middle class features a strong reliance on educational attainment (the ownership of expertise) for much of its social and economic well-being. The following chart further explains the strong correlation between educational attainment and personal as well as household income: that as education goes up, annual income goes up. Table 4.1 shows the increases in income for groups of adults as their education levels rises.

Muennig (2006) made the connection when he found empirically that "each student who graduates from high school [not to mention college] instead of dropping out before getting a high school diploma will save states an average of $13,706 (in 2005 dollars) in Medicaid and expenditures for uninsured care over the course of his or her lifetime" (p. 43). When we multiply the health costs for dropouts, by the number of them, we see a powerful example of the connection between education, health care, and costs to society.

The Alliance for Excellence in Education concluded that "if the approximately 1.2 million young people who were estimated to drop out of school in the United States this year could earn diplomas, states could save more than $17 billion over the course of those young people's lifetimes. Furthermore, similar savings at national and local levels could accrue for every class of high school students who graduate rather than drop out, producing an annual repetition and boon to our nation's coffers" (Alliance for Excellence in Education, Policy Brief, 2006, p. 1).

Hence, going on to college and graduating mean higher incomes, less dependence on public health programs such as Medicare, and access to

Table 4.1 Median and Individual Income and Education Level

Criteria		Overall	Less than ninth grade	High school dropout	High school graduate	Some college	Associates degree	Bachelor's degree	Bachelor's degree or more	Master's degree	Professional degree	Doctoral degree
Median individual income	Male, age 25+	$33,517	$15,461	$18,990	$28,763	$35,073	$39,015	$50,916	$55,751	$61,698	$88,530	$73,853
	Female, age 25+	$19,679	$9,296	$10,786	$15,962	$21,007	$24,808	$31,309	$35,125	$41,334	$48,536	$53,003
Median household income		$45,016	$18,787	$22,718	$36,835	$45,854	$51,970	$68,728	$73,446	$78,541	$100,000	$96,830

better medical care. The Alliance for Excellent Education, with support from the MetLife Foundation, reached the following conclusions in their study of Health, Wealth, and Education (2006):

- *People with lower educational attainment have less insurance coverage*: 4.5 million or almost 16 percent of the US population has no coverage (US Census Bureau, 2006), as those with less education are "considerably less likely to have health coverage."
- *Individuals who lack health insurance receive less medical care and have poorer health:* Even adults with chronic illnesses, according to Davidoff and Kenny (2005), are "less likely to receive care and necessary prescriptions than insured adults."

   So not only would the government save money on health care, but individuals would also earn more money, live better lives, contribute more to society—and their children would benefit into the next generation.
- *Education leads to healthier lives.* Besides giving families better access to good health care, "better educated people are able to follow doctors' instructions successfully and to navigate medical bureaucracy" (p. 4). While better educated people often get cleaner, healthier jobs, those with lower levels of education attainment often work in less healthier environments with more hazardous chemicals and machines (Winkelby et al., 1992, p. 818)

Changing Together

We do see some changes in health care and education, although improvements are moving slowly. Public education has become more "privatized" with greater family choice and mobility, as students receive state vouchers to attend private and even religious schools—legal under *Zelman v. Simmons-Harris* (2002), a court case originating in Ohio after the state passed a voucher law that was implemented mainly in Cleveland.

   Some states now gives vouchers to the poorest families who can enroll their children in religiously affiliated private and charter schools, a practice that the high court declared legal, since parents made the final enrollment decision, not the government. And public schools are offering more choice "within the system," using "magnet schools" (Cooper, 1987), open enrollment, and other local and regional option. And it's now legal in most states to keep a child home for "home-schooling" (Cooper, 2005), a choice that was illegal and uncommon until recent years.

And we see public support for charter schools, which are "privately" owned and run schools, sometimes affiliated with a religious foundation or group. Thus, education is privatizing and giving greater options and choice, while the health-care system is become more public, through Medicare and Medicaid, for older and sicker patients who are poor. So while sick persons with funds can chose their physicians and clinics, poor families with kids can determine with boundaries which school to select, and whether to enter a lottery to win a voucher to "pay their way into" their school of choice. Whichever services they seek in health care and education, their levels of choice are both related in a number of ways to family wealth and income.

Learning from the Education and Health Connection

What can health and education do to improve, in a sense learn from, each other? Five things:

1. Making Good Education and Health Care
Available to Rich and Poor

Both services should be affordable and available, health care like education! Education is readily and widely available, and all children attend schools; meanwhile health services are more scattered, and can be more costly. So only the elderly and the very poor get Medicare and Medicaid coverage. And the middle- and lower-middle classes can hardly afford it, unless they work for a company or public agency that provides health care as a work benefit.

A study (Woodhandler et al., 2003) comparing the costs of administering health care in the United States and Canada shows some amazing results. Besides not extending health care to all, the United States spends more on running the limited system than Canada does.

Canada as shown below in Table 4.2 has a more socialized medical system, and much lower overhead in managing the service. In US dollars, in 1999, the United States has more limited health services that are more expensive to insure, manage, administer, and run, per capita in US dollars. So while the US system is less comprehensive, it is also more inefficient to run.

President Obama has proposed a form of universal health care that provides universal, available, and portable health care for all. As the *New York Times* (March 23, 2010) announced, "With the strokes of 22 pens, President Obama signed his landmark health care overhaul—the most

Table 4.2   Costs of Health-care Administration in the United States and Canada, 1999

Cost Category	Spending per Capita ($) UNITED STATES	Spending per Capita ($) CANADA
Insurance overhead	$259	$47
Employers' costs to manage health benefits	57	8
Hospital administration	315	103
Nursing home administration	62	29
Administrative costs of practitioners	324	107
Home care administration	42	13
TOTAL	$1059	$307

expansive social legislation enacted in decades—into law on Tuesday, saying it enshrines 'the core principle that everybody should have some basic security when it comes to their health care." Thus, Obama's ideas would modernize the system to lower costs and improve quality, and third, the plan promotes preventative services and strengthens health care.

2. Both Services Should Be Based on Choice and the Needs of Users, Like Free Medical Care and Some Charter Schools, Vouchers, and Scholarships to Private Schools

As we see, schools are becoming more diverse, more privatized: for example, states are offering vouchers to families in cities such as Milwaukee and Cleveland that allow parents to select from a range of private and religious schools (Catholic, Lutheran, Jewish, and Seventh-day Adventist)—and the public funds "follow" the child to the school. Why not give every child a voucher, worth around $12,000 (the national average per pupil spending for public schooling), and let parents and their children decide on a school that meets their needs?

The money would follow the child to the school. And the child would likely have a better chance of graduating, going on to college, and earning a good living. Those very poor parents, living in Los Angeles, who were able to gain scholarships to Catholic schools did much better than their public school counterparts, as Archbishop Gomez (2011) in *Education Week* reported:

> A recent study on the impact of Catholic schools in the lives of economically disadvantaged children found that 98 percent of a group of low-income students attending Catholic schools on tuition grants in Los Angeles

graduated high school. What's more, nearly 98 percent of them went on to pursue some sort of post-secondary education, the same study, done by the School of Education at Loyola Marymount University. (*Education Week*, www.edweek.org/ew, p. 4)

While this sample of students is hardly random, we do see a strong connection between lower and higher education among a small cohort of Catholic school students. And in New York City, even for Rice High School, a Catholic secondary school that closed for lack of funds, a report showed that all the graduates were accepted to college.

And starting better schooling earlier with better programs can make a lifetime of differences. As the Task Force appointed by the Economic Policy Institute found in "A Broader, Bolder Approach to Education" (see Noguera, 2011), medical services could learn much from the public school system, which is organized to provide schooling for all. Somewhere between the public (socialist) and private (market) models of public provision, a "golden mean" must be found: where good health makes better education possible and also improves education; and education, as we know it, enables high school and college graduates to make a better living and raise their children with more opportunities, and better health and education—the connections are here.

In an effort to mitigate the effects of poverty, Pedro A. Noguera (2011, p. 11) explains the opportunities and limitations of schools:

> While expecting a single school to counter the effects of poverty on its own is unrealistic, a small but growing number of American schools are finding ways to reduce some of the effects. Mitigation is not needs of children. A growing body of research shows that when schools can offer students access to a variety of social services (e.g., licensed social workers or psychologists, nurse practitioners, or dental services), academic and developmental outcomes for children can improve. (Darling-Hammond, 2010, p.11)

3. Both Should Be Closely Monitored to Improve Medical Practices, and School Instruction and Programs

Since both education and health care are vital human services, we need better information of who's using the systems, what services they are receiving, and how effectively the education and medical care are being delivered (Anderson et al., 2005). In what ways and where are people healthier and better educated? We have the data scattered at different levels and in different jurisdictions (federal, state, and local), as this chapter has shown, on progress in health, and education delivery and effects.

But key leaders, and groups of families, need to help collect, analyze, and share the results, all to show how best to get educated and healthier.

Further, what we're trying to do now as a society, is track the processes, and long-term effects as well as the effectiveness of education and health provision. We know that they are linked, and we know that they must begin early (earlier): health care before birth and education soon thereafter.

For example, "Broader and Bolder Approaches," a publication notes that "research supports the provision of prenatal care for all pregnant women, and preventative and routine pediatric, dental, and optometric care for all infants, toddlers, and schoolchildren, to minimize the extent to which health problems become obstacles to success in school" (Noguera, 2011, p. 5).

Thus, health-care services should be monitored, along with academic development and growth, since the two are related, which would require the changing and augmenting of health coverage and help. Accountability must be broadened, expanded to look at the child, the family, and community, and to provide and evaluate the needs of the children from birth to adulthood. As the bolder approach recognizes:

> Weakening the link between social [e.g., medical] and economic disadvantages and low-income achievement—leaving no child behind—is an urgent priority. With our population aging and schools serving a growing number of disproportionately aging and immigrant children, the future viability of our education, health and other social institutions will be affected by how well we educate young people of all background. (p. 7)

Thus, not only is poor education and health going to affect the next generation, but this connection between schooling and medical care will also have an impact on the older generation who are dependent on social security and other services. One generation affects the other!

In addition, research indicates, interestingly, that GP (general practitioners) believe in a national survey that health care should be provided to all children, while "specialists" are less willing. The Jackson Healthcare Survey in 2010 found that physician's political views on the plan [Obama's health plan] from the American Medical Association does reform the US health care effectively. The Jackson survey concluded that "physician respondents, the majority of whom considered themselves knowledgeable or very knowledgeable about the act, gave PPACA [Patient Protection and Affordable Care Act] an average grade of D." The secretary of Health and Human Service, Kathleen Sebelius, concluded that "the premiums would be too high and healthy people would not sign up" (*New York Times*, Pear, October 15, 2011, p. 1).

4. Both Education and Health Should and Are Developing and Using the Latest, Best Technology to Improve Services, Practices, and Programs

Technology is here to stay, and pervades every aspect of life. Microsurgery in hospitals is an example, as men with cancer can have their prostate gland removed using a microsurgery equipment called "a Di Vinci surgical device." And teachers are learning to Skype a lesson or seminar in education to attach students to each other and to the world of knowledge online.

As one source explained (http://en.wikipedia.org/wiki/Skype):

> Skype in the classroom is a free global community that invites teachers to collaborate on classroom projects where they might use Skype, and share skills and inspiration around specific teaching needs. Teachers all over the world are using Skype to make learning more exciting and memorable. It's easy to see why: Skype offers an immediate way to help students discover new cultures, languages and ideas, all without leaving the classroom.

5. Both Should Be Readily Available and Accessible to All Americans, as a Key Way to Improve Their Lives, Help Them Grow and Be Well, and Contribute to the Society: With Income, Productivity, Creativity, and Well-Being

It's never easy to succeed: when schools do, they may be criticized by competing schools for doing better and attracting more and better students. For example, when the leading school in New York State (and New York City) wanted to open a branch on the fancy Upper West Side of New York City, the public school leaders fought the idea, for fear of greater competition. One dramatic urban case, under the leadership of politician, Evan Moscowitz, was her attempt to move the Harlem Success Academy into a fancy neighborhood in New York City. There again, the local schools feared the competition,

Charters Raise the School-Performance Tide

Despite all the good she's done—her Harlem Success Academy 1 ranks in the top percentile of schools in New York State, and the others in the network are no slouches—Eva Moskowitz has earned herself some fierce opponents among Gotham's upper-middle class. How come? First, a year ago, she sought to locate one of her schools on the Upper West Side—only to see hordes of public-school parents freak out at the thought of their schools competing with a new charter for space, money, and kids. (After some effort, Moskowitz opened the school this fall.)…As Moscowitz (2009) has explained, "middle-class families need options, too." (p. 12)

Little doubt now: good schools are attracted to good neighborhoods, with middle-class families to support them. But good schools, in good neighborhoods may help to equalize educational opportunity. And free or subsidized medical services, disease prevention, and fast, available health procedures will mean a longer, better life. While all of these services are interconnected, we know too that good education and health relate and promote better jobs and high family incomes.

The Alliance for Excellent Education (2006) sums up the critical relations among the three factors: education, wealth, and health as follows:

States could save $17 billion nationally, a savings that could be earned for each class of students who graduate high school rather than drop out. This potential public benefit is just one among a multitude of positive results that would accrue to society if America's educational system successfully educated *all* of its citizens—instead of allowing over a million youth to drop out without a diploma each year. A citizenry that is not only healthier, but also wealthier and wiser, is an asset that every state, and the country as a whole, needs. (p. 4)

References

Alliance for Excellent Education (2006). *Straight A's: Public Education Policy and Progress. Policy Brief. 6*(23), 33.

Anderson, G., Hussey, P. S., Frogner, B. K., & Waters, H. R. (2005). Health spending in the United States and the rest of the industrialized world. *Health Affairs, 24*(4), 903–914.

Cooper, B. S. (2005). *Home schooling in full view.* Greenwich, CT: Information Age Publishing.

———. (1987). *Magnet Schools.* London: Institute of Economic Affairs.

Darling-Hammond, L. (2010). *The flat world and education: How America's commitment to equity will determine our future.* New York: Teachers College Press.

Davidoff, A., & Kenny, G. (2005). *Uninsured Americans with chronic health conditions: Key findings from the National Health Survey.* Washington, DC: Urban Institute.

Department of Health and Human Services (2009). National Health Expenditures Data www.cms.gov/Research-Statistics-Data. *Washington, DC: Center for Medicare & Medicaid Services.*

Federal Interagency Forum on Child and Family Statistics (2011). *America's children: Key national indicators of well-being, 2011.* Washington, DC: US Government Printing Office.

Fussel, Paul. (1997). *Class: A guide through the American status system.* New York: Touchstone

Gilbert, D. (1997). *American class structure in an age of growing inequality.* New York: Wadsworth.

Hadley, J. (2003). *Sicker and poorer: The consequences of being uninsured.* Washington, DC: Urban Institute.

Kaiser Family Foundation (2007, September), *Health insurance premiums rise 6.1 percent in 2007.* Washington, DC: Health Research and Education Trust.

Levine, R. (1998). *Social class and stratification.* Lanham, MD: Rowman & Littlefield.

Moscowitz, E. (2009). *Harlem success academy.* New York: New York Times.

Muennig, P. (2006). *State-level health cost-savings associated with improvements in high school graduation rates.* Washington, DC: A report commissioned by the Alliance for Excellence in Education.

Noguera, P. S. (2011, October 27*). A broader and bolder approach uses education to break the cycle of poverty. Phi Delta Kappan, 11.*

Pierce v. Society of Sisters of the Holy Names of Jesus and Mary, 268 US 510 (1925).

Robey, P. (2011). *Catholic schools and educating the whole child.* Education Week. Retrieved from www.edweek.org/ew.

US Census Bureau (2006). Health Insurance Status by Age, Race, Hispanic Origin and Income. U.S. Department of Congress.

Winkelby, M., Jatulis, D., Frank, E., & Fortmann, S. (1992). Socioeconomic status and health: How education, income, and occupation contribute to risk factor for cardiovascular disease. *American Journal of Public Health, 82*(6), 816–820.

Woodhandler, S., Campbell, T., & Himmelsetein, M. H. A. (2003). Costs of health care management in the USA and Canada. *New England Journal of Medicine, 49,* 768–775.

Zelman v. Simmons-Harris (2002). 536 U.S. 639.

5

Connecting Good Health Care to Educational Attainment

Introduction

Becoming educated requires consistency in school attendance, the ability to concentrate, and a sense of confidence in one's academic success. Students, unable to receive adequate and preventative health care often fail in school, as they may be absent more often, be less able to concentrate, and lack clear focus on instruction and learning. This chapter connects good health care—or bad—to educational achievement or lack thereof—conditions that appear to be perpetuated from generation to generation.

For example, recent reports from the US Center for Disease Control (2010) indicate that 59 million Americans have no health care nor access to preventative medical service that could likely curtail serious physical and/or psychological conditions, and/ or premature death. As Dr. Thomas Frieden (2010) reported, "Both adults and kids have lost private coverage over the last decade" (n.p.).

In particular, according to the Children's Defense Fund and Policy Priorities (2010), some 8.1 million children are uninsured; and a half-million pregnant women have no medical coverage, creating the possibility of delivering children with low birth-weight and other medical complications, negatively affecting infants before they begin their lives.

People who receive little or no health care are sicker and die sooner. Undiagnosed and untreated illnesses, and poorly managed health care, greatly increase the child's frequency of debilitating physical and mental diseases. Researchers from the Johns Hopkins Children's Center analyzed data from 38 states on hospitalization, and death rates of children with no health-care services from 1988 to 2005.

The alarming statistic from the Johns Hopkins Children's Center study revealed that uninsured American children faced a 60 percent greater risk of dying than those children covered by health care. Adding to this disturbing result is that children who are dying enter the hospital in crisis and die within 24 hours of admittance—as nothing could be done to save them.

Relating Health to Learning

Chronic absences in the early years of schooling have a lasting impact on students' educational success; opportunities for sustainable employment; and/or the prerequisite for adequate support to family, community, and society. Early grades in school set the foundation for learning in all subject areas. Literacy and mathematical principles underlie proficiency for more complex learning in later grades. Missing these educational foundations and skills, due to poor health and health care, can have profound negative outcomes for future success. The lack of routine care and preventive measures is a major problem in the United States, as our healthcare system is still basically fee-charging and based on employment health care, which can affect the poor and unemployed adults and their families.

How do poor health and lack of adequate nutrition and well-being affect young people's ability to learn? Abraham Maslow, in 1954, identified the needs of all human beings to reach their individual potentials. His philosophy remains a constant in physiological and cognitive development for children and their ability to learn. In his research, Maslow countered the philosophy that motivation depended on birth and biology and posited his idea on two prime reasons: deficiency and needs.

Thus, students who are deficient in the following have greater difficulty in achieving in school and completing the courses of study necessary for graduation and academic advancement:

1) *Physiological well-being*: avoiding hunger, thirst, bodily discomforts, etc.;
2) *Safety/security*: being out of danger;
3) *Belongingness and love*: affiliate with others, be accepted; and
4) *Esteem*: to achieve, be competent, gain approval and recognition.

According to Maslow, each of the needs, from 1 to 4 above, must be met sequentially for a person to become *self-actualized*. The ability to become self-actualized, to problem solve, appreciate opportunities offered in life, and continue to grow personally and socially is dependent on one's schooling and success. People who are at lowest level of Maslow's scale are interested only in coping and surviving from one day to the next. Seeking knowledge to empower oneself either economically or socially is not important or receives no thought or effort.

Students—who are absent for more than 10 days in a 180-day-school year because of physiological illness or who are present in school but lethargic due to feeling unwell—become defeated in their effort to learn. As Barbara Wolf (1999) explains, "The issue of the links between poverty, health and access to medical care...has received considerable attention from a variety of perspectives. Health influences most activities of life, from the ability to engage in learning to the ability to enjoy life itself" (p. 9).

Poor health affects school performance in many ways. Absenteeism results in lack of continuity in knowledge-building that is necessary for each step on the educational ladder. Poor concentration due to feeling ill, weak or tired, and hungry has an effect on concentration or the ability to participate in the classroom or extracurricular activities. According to one study, students who miss more than 10 days in a 90-day semester have difficulty remaining on grade level.

In a report on children with chronic poor health entitled, *The Influence of Health on School Outcomes*, Wolf (1985) found that absenteeism in general is associated with lower achievement in school (measured by achievement groupings based on standardized test scores). She also found that absenteeism due to chronic illness is related to an even lower achievement in school than the general high absence, due to insufficient energy and a general feeling a malaise.

Children in poor families are likely to do worse in school than those who reside in nonpoor families, studies have indicated. Poor children, according to a report by state university.com, are twice as likely to have repeated a grade in school or been suspended or expelled due to behavior and disruptions. Examining the number of referrals and identification for learning difficulties, children from impoverished homes seem to fill the limits for special education classes as compared to children who have better health, attendance, and concentration.

Lack of health care due to poverty has the greatest effect on a child's early life and schooling when foundations of learning are being taught. Educational outcomes for young children are dependent on the following:

- Health and nutrition
- Parental support and relationships

- Neighborhood conditions that support health and safety
- School quality for resources, class size, experienced teachers, and childcare facilities.

Studies have found that children who reside in deep poverty have no health care, and are absent more often score ten to twelve point lower on standardized tests measuring achievement and cognitive abilities than those who live in simply low-income households. A study by Linda Pagani (1999), "found that persistent poverty was significantly related to academic failure. Children who had experienced poverty throughout their lives were twice as likely as never-poor children to be placed in a non-age appropriate classroom" (p. 3).

Lack of Learning Readiness

Findings concerning the affect of poverty and health-care issues go beyond early childhood. The long-term consequences of poor health are directly related to cognitive and academic outcomes in not only early, but also middle and late childhood. Failures become cumulative and dropout from school is too often the result. Longitudinal studies have found that the developmental outcomes of children raised in poverty suffer due to lack in both academic and physiological readiness. As poor children enter school in kindergarten, language development is half that of their non-poor counterparts. The deficiency compounds as standards are not met and failure becomes the rule of the day.

The research on the lack of health care for poor families finds that mothers who have little or no prenatal care are 80 percent more likely to have babies with low birth-weight indices than that of their nonpoor counterparts. Children with low birth-weights tend to have more health problems throughout childhood. According to a study done by Smith, Fauth, and Gunn (1996), "compared to full-term children, neurologically intact very low-birth-weight children present more impairments in arithmetic, motor and spatial skills, language and memory, and perform worse on measures of achievement" (p. 39). Some studies indicate that the detrimental effects of prenatal neglect and low birth weight remain a constant inhibitor to learning throughout the adolescent and adult years.

Table 5.1 shows the difference in readiness between students who live in poverty and those who do not. Kindergarten readiness is the basis for success in later grades, and with current standards and earlier grade expectations for learning, the impact is even more distressing.

Table 5.1   Readiness and SES

Beginning Kindergarten Students' Readiness Skills by Socioeconomic Status	Lowest SES	Highest SES
Recognizing Letters of the Alphabet	39%	85%
Identifying Beginning Sounds of Words	10%	51%
Identifying Primary Colors	69%	90%
Counting to 20	48%	68%
Writing Own Name	54%	76%
Amount of Time Read to Prior to Kindergarten	25 Hours	1,000 Hours
Accumulated Experience with Words	13 Million Words	45 Million Words

Source: Adapted from Low and Burkham (2002). Copyright 2002 by Economic Policy Institute.

The differences noted stem not only from the lack of resources, books, and experiences to prepare children for school, but also from poor beginnings in health that detract from the possibility to do well in the academic arenas for learning.

School performance can be judged on many levels, from resources to teacher qualification to community support. One thing is abundantly clear: school performance correlates with attendance and engagement in the classroom. The US Department of Education correlates school success with readiness to learn. And as early as 1990, the year that the National Education Goals were established, the department stated, "Children will receive the nutrition and health care needed to arrive at school with healthy minds and bodies" (Zill, 1990, p. 2).

Poor health means less of opportunity to learn: sick, distracted, labeled, retained, absent, and malnourished; living unhealthy lives undercuts the child's ability to think, concentrate, and learn. Sick kids have more trouble learning—and it gets worse!

Health as a Community Concern

Home and community environments contributing to poor health often go uninvestigated by agencies responsible for health and safety. Living conditions in tenements, apartments, and unsafe single-family dwellings expose children to asbestos, and lead-painted woodwork is a major concern in the cognitive and physical development of young children. Elevated blood levels in children living in poor neighborhoods and asbestos-related lung disease in poor housing are four times greater than those living in less-impoverished homes. Results from exposure may include stunted growth, lower cognitive ability, lung disease, and other various illnesses and physical impairments.

Emergency rooms are overcrowded in poor neighborhoods and locations where residents have little or no health care. As indicated, emergency rooms for emergency care only are the primary resource for many when they are well along in their illness or injury. The lack of preventive care and the use of the emergency room when illness is further along, contribute to the overall issue of health, education, and welfare. Children are the most susceptible and more die often, having had little preventive care for childhood diseases. According to Dr. Peter J. Pronovost (2009), "The striking thing is that children (who have adequate health care) don't often die. The study provides further evidence that the need to insure everyone is a moral issue, not just an economic one" (*New York Times,* October 30, 2009).

About 14.1 million children living in the United States, statistically 1 in 5, are living on or below the poverty line. Poor children, who are less healthy, lag behind their nonpoor peers emotionally, physically, and in intellectual development. The problems continue to accumulate throughout their lifetimes, perpetuating lack of achievement, poor health, and inability to move beyond their current circumstances. The most common causes for children to be hospitalized are from complications at birth, asthma, and pneumonia. These conditions are present in many children, but the outcomes are far different depending on the child's health-care status.

Poverty, Oral Health, and Learning

We have all experienced the visit to the dentist. It is estimated that 90 percent of the population from young childhood through 64 years of age has had tooth decay or cavities in need of treatment. Tooth decay is one of the most common diseases in childhood and untreated, contributes to pain and oral infections. Children living in poverty suffer more tooth decay than their nonpoor counterparts. They are less likely to receive the preventative treatments protecting teeth, affecting their abilities' to achieve in the academic setting.

Surgeon General David Satcher (2001) explains, when a child's oral health is neglected, their ability to learn is impacted. He emphasizes, "What amounts to a silent epidemic of dental and oral diseases is affecting some population groups. This burden of disease restricts activities in schools, work and home, and often significantly diminishes the quality of life."

In the report, Satcher indicated that approximately 51-million-school hours per year are lost due to dental and oral-related illnesses. Adults with chronic tooth pain and oral disease are more likely to miss work, and due to tooth loss eat foods that are easily swallowed but less nutritious.

Often overlooked as a chronic problem, oral health care affects all components of life and needs to be an integral part of the community health-care design. Health outcomes relative to poor neighborhoods and communities are starkly different than outcomes in middle to affluent areas. The United States, according to Karen Stripp (2010), "the nation with the world's largest gross domestic product watches more of its babies die, and more young adults die than any other nation in the group of seven (G7) industrialized countries (United Kingdom, Canada, Japan, Germany, Italy and France)" (p. 1).

The economic shift, the loss of jobs, and health care has produced a new "poor" in the country. The situation has changed the lives of many who were once independent and considered middle class. The new poor along with the persistent has increased the number of children living in poor and near-poor families. And, research continues to show that relatively poor children develop more physical and cognitive disparities in comparison to children who live in middle and affluent environments.

A 1997 Harvard study found that the life expectancy for people living in poor neighborhoods was lower than those residing in more-affluent communities by as much as 15 years. And while poor health due to lack of preventive care is certainly a factor, an overlooked cause is the pollution that exists from various environmental sources.

A study prepared for the California State Waste Management Board, known as the "Cerrell Report," concluded that "trash incinerators should not be built within five miles of middle and higher socioeconomic strata neighborhoods." The report, "Political Difficulties Facing Waste-to-Energy Conversion Plant Siting," says, "that plans to build such plants will face less opposition if placed in poor neighborhoods instead of wealthy ones. The report provides personality profiles of people most likely and least likely to fight an incineration plant" (Olden, 1998, p. 7).

And, in a Public Broadcasting System documentary (2008) focusing on poor health in communities, the following conditions were pervasive and obvious:

- Low social and economic status
- Pervasive poverty in families and group dwellings
- Apparent racism
- Immigration status and exclusion
- Oppression
- Neighborhood blight and violence.

Thus, in communities where the poor reside and financial resources are limited, choices for housing, schools, and clinics for health care are inadequate, compounding and perpetuating physical health and cognitive development. Brady-Smith, Fauth, and Gunn (1996) summarize, "Financial strain limits the housing and neighborhood choices...constraining these families to live in neighborhoods characterized by high levels of crime and unemployment, low levels of resources and a lack of collective efficacy among residents." (p. 39)

Parenting, Families, and Perpetuation

Economic stress, poor living conditions, and nutritional deficiencies lead to parenting that is less consistent, harsher, more punitive and less involved in the daily needs of young children through the adolescent and teenage years. Without physical and emotional support and guidance, children young and older too often fail in school and drop out before skills or training can be completed, perpetuating low-income jobs, poverty, and despair.

Exacerbating the problem is the number of single-parent households contributing to the lack of income and time involved in a child's upbringing. Brooks-Gunn (2001) comments, "Single-parent families are more likely to be poor due to their dependence on a single wage earner and the probability that the household heads are younger and less educated than their dual-parent counterparts...it is not surprising that 53 percent of poor families are headed by solely a female adult" (p. 181).

Mothers, who have had unsuccessful educational experiences, have had no mentoring from their own mothers, and who struggle in their daily existence tend to neglect their own children perpetuating the cycle of failure. In an e! Science News report, social competence and behavior problems in children are often observed as early as kindergarten. Researchers Dr. Alice C. Carter and colleagues (2010) examined the relationship of sociodemographics with aberrant psychosocial behaviors and found that children (21.6 percent) born into these circumstances were more likely to suffer from varying forms of psychopathology in the early pre- and early-school-aged years. Dr. Carter et al. (2010) reported,

> Socio-demographic and psychosocial correlates included persistent poverty beginning in early childhood, limited parental education, low family expressiveness, stressful life events, and violence exposure. Finally, diagnostic status was significantly associated with poorer social competence and family burden. (n.p.)

Mental health problems seen in schools are often misdiagnosed as behavior problems, and instead of receiving the care necessary for the family and the child, a special education setting becomes the outcome. Maternal mental health becomes a perpetuating force and is negatively influenced by family stress, low education, and inability to cope with the demands of children. Children are affected in their cognitive abilities to concentrate, and experience academic underachievement, aggressiveness toward peers, and finally suspension from school. And so it continues from one generation to the next...

The Value of Preventative Care

Chronic diseases are the most common of all health problems in children and young adults. These illnesses are also the most preventable and would be less costly to society by improving human capital for employment, self-sustenance, academic achievement, and contribution to society as a whole. Routine prenatal physical examinations for young mothers prevent low-birth weights and the physical and cognitive problems associated with it. Routine physical examinations of young children can minimize the effects of childhood diseases and prevent complications.

Doctors and clinics can advise young mothers on how to manage nutritional menus and supplements for healthy growth: physically, emotionally, and academically. Physicians can be part of an education process to support healthy practices, empower parents to take responsibility for preventative care, and manage daily routines to promote healthy living. The lack of facilities for parents to access doctors, dentists, and clinic has long and deleterious effects on the entire community and the whole of society.

Summary

Connections of good health care to learning are profound and evident. The effect of poverty and poor health care can be seen in national, state, and local statistics. National mandates for testing, while controversial, do tell a significant story when connecting health, physical, mental, and cognitive statuses to scores and community wealth.

The effect of poverty on children's mental and physical health begins early on and continues through adolescence and adulthood. Absenteeism, academic underachievement, placement in special education settings, suspensions, and dropouts are all connected to health and education. Children who are raised in poverty and suffer the consequences of chronic disease, poor oral health, community pollution, and family stresses, face adverse developmental outcomes in the home, school, and community.

Statistically, 26 percent of the US population falls in the age range of 18 and under. Yet, of that 26 percent, 40 percent live in poverty. Connecting poor health care, substandard education, and community blight to the outcomes reported on state and national statistics, the evidence is clear: health, education, and welfare are the links for success or likely failure.

Without health, school success is unlikely; without health, employment is unsustainable; and without health, well-being in the home and community impossible. Families who live in high-poverty areas with few resources are likely to remain in a quagmire of perpetuation from generation to generation.

References

Brady-Smith, C. B., Fauth, R. C., & Brooks-Gunn, J. (1996). "The consequences of living in poverty for young children's cognitive and verbal ability and early school achievement." In G. J. Duncan, & J. Brooks-Gunn (Eds.), *Consequences of growing up poor* (pp. 37–45). New York: Russell Sage.

Brooks-Gunn, J. (2001). Effects of combining public assistance and employment on young mothers and their children. *Women and Health,* 32, 179–201.

Carter, L. C. (2010 July 8). Science News. Retrieved from http://esciencenews.com/articles/2010/07/1.5.preschoolers.us.demonstrates.mental.health.issues.when.entering.kindergarten.

Children's Defense Fund and Policy Priorities. (2010). Retrieved from www.childrensdefense.org/policy- priorities.

Frieden, Dr. Thomas, director of the US Centers for Disease Control and Prevention. (2010, March 16). In a news briefing, *New York Times.*

Low, V., & Burkham, D. (2002). Economic Policy Institute. In S. Neuman & D. Dickinson (Eds.), *Handbook of early literacy research* (pp. 121–132). Boston: Guilford Press.

Maslow, A. (1954). Retrieved from www.abraham-maslow.com.

Olden, K. (1998). The complex interaction of poverty, pollution, health status." *The Scientist* 12(4): 7.

Pagani, L. (1999). *Poverty and education- overview, children and adolescents.* Retrieved from http://education.stateuuniversity.com/pages/2330/Poverty-Education.html.

Pronovost, Dr. P. J. (2009, October 30). Hospitalized children without health insurance are more likely to die.*New York Times.*

Public Broadcasting System Documentary (2008, April 2). *Unnatural Causes: Is inequity making us sick?*

Satcher, Surgeon General. (2001, March 5) US Public Health Service Department of Health and Human Services. Statement at Special Hearing before the US Senate Committee on Appropriations. Anchorage, AK.

Stripp, K. (2010, November 9). Poor health and social inequity: A reflection on the US class system. In *Cultural Expressions Magazine, 32*, 1. Social Welfare Research, University of Kansas. US Center for Disease Control Report.

Wolf, B. L. (1999, September). Poverty, children's health, and health care utilization. *FRBNY Economic Policy Review*, 9.

———. (1985). The influence of health on school outcomes: A multivariate approach. *Medical Care, 23*(10), 127–138.

Zill, N. (1990). *Child health and school readiness: Background paper on national educational goals.* Washington DC: Child Trends Inc., 2.

6

Education Relates to Income and Life-Chances

Clearly associations abound between quality of life, physical health, psychological well-being, and the education of parents and their children. Positive environments—consisting of a supportive home life, good health care, and appropriate schooling—create better connections to self, home, community, and beyond. As Robert Denis Mare (1995) explains:

> As the economic rewards of education continue to increase, so too do the numbers of people in the United States with degrees and credentials. With an increasing number of adults returning to school and young people making choices about education, it is valuable to know more about earnings and degrees. (p. 156)

This chapter explores the education-income relationship from both ends: first, how educational opportunities and quality are affected by the background and income (wealth) of parents and the communities in which they live. And, we examine how educational levels relate to personal income, starting right after college, continuing through mid-career, and over a lifetime. And finally, we examine society's education as a predictor of a nation's long-term development and prosperity. For as Alan Greenspan, former leader of the Federal Reserve System, explained :

> Even the most significant advances in information and technology will not produce additional economic value without human creativity and intellect...the U.S. system of education must remain the world's leader in generating scientific and technological breakthroughs and in preparing workers to meet the need for skilled labor...Education must realize the potential for bringing lasting benefits to the economy. (Romboy, 2000, p. D6)

Money thus works both ways: helping students to get a good education, and often providing the means to earn higher income from being well-educated, making them better consumers and higher taxpayers! And the collective effect of good education and improved earnings is an improved economy and industry. And a poor education can mean the opposite. Thus, we hear the warnings:

> If current trends continue, the proportion of workers with high school diplomas and college degrees will decrease and the personal income of Americans will decline over the next 15 years. Substantial increases in those segments of America's young population with the lowest level of education, combined with the coming retirement of the baby boomers—the most highly educated generation in U.S. history—are projected to lead to a drop in the average level of education of the U.S. workforce over the next two decades, unless states do a better job of raising the educational level of all racial/ethnic groups. (Youniss and Convey, 2004, p. 25)

A child's welfare is thus directly affected by the conditions at home, school, and the doctor's. Each is a determinant of growth and development, sustainability, and reliance. Research shows that families with resources can usually find a good education for their children, in several ways,—regardless of their children's needs, talents, and expectations—in several ways. Funding and supporting good public, private and religious education constitute the substance of this chapter to further education for all students, regardless of background—first language and level of family income. We show that wealth and income are related to education, in complex ways. More income can give parents more education options for their children; and a good education can open job and career options that in turn can often mean higher income.

Starting Families Later and Later

Research shows that one of the most dramatic effects of changes in society, education, and in employment is that marriages and childrearing are starting later and later in the lives of Americans. For example, Frank F. Furstenberg (2010) found that home-leaving, marriage, and the onset of childbearing take place much later in the life span than they did during the period following World War II. He explains the "longer" and "later" as follows:

> After the disappearance of America's well-paying unskilled and semi-skilled manufacturing jobs during the 1960s, youth from all economic strata began remaining in school longer and marrying and starting their

own families later. Increasing numbers of lower-income women did not marry at all but chose, instead, non-marital parenthood—often turning to their natal families for economic and social support, rather than to their partners. (p. 44)

Changes in family structure and work can have an effect on children, as they are now typically born later to the parents, and the mother and/or father may be heavily engrossed in work and careers by the time the baby is born.

And we don't pay much attention to our younger adults, who without their parents and relatives, have little ready resources, as their work is just starting and the expenses (housing, jobs, training, and travel) are high. Thus, Furstenberg further (2010) reports:

Unlike many nations in Europe, the United States, with its relatively underdeveloped welfare system, does not invest heavily in education, health care, and job benefits for young adults. It relies, instead, on families' investments in their own adult children. But as the transition to adulthood becomes more protracted, the increasing family burden may prove costly to society as a whole. (p. 43)

Education and Income

Relating education level to income is a complex process, as some well-educated people, with doctorates such as the authors of this book, have elected to teach university, and often earn less than the folks with a BA who go into business and commerce. But the averages are quite clear: with each leap up the education "ladder," weekly mean (average) income goes up, as presented in Table 6.1 from the *Occupation Outlook Quarter* in

Table 6.1   Median Income Weekly for Full-Time Wage/Salary Workers, 25 or Older, 2005

Educational Level	Earning Per Week
Doctoral Degree	$ 1,421
Professional Degree	$ 1,370
Master's Degree	$ 1,129
Bachelor's Degree	$ 937
Associate Degree	$ 699
National Medium Income Per Week	**$ 696**
Some college, no degree	$ 653
High school, no college	$ 583
Less than high school diploma	$ 409

2006 that shows weekly income in 2005 by degrees with the average being almost $700 per week, the top at $1,421, and the least income for those without degrees at about $400 weekly income.

Of course, both apprenticeships and on-the-job training can help to upgrade skills and increase workers' incomes, where high-tech workers such as machinists and electricians can earn as much per week as college graduates. And besides calculating weekly median incomes, research-ers have also compared "life-time earning streams" and find enormous differences between those with college degrees and beyond, versus those with a high school diploma or less.

Thus, the hunt for a good, affordable available education for children is many families' major effort with many options and different levels of cost.

Finding a Good School

1. *Better Housing and High Quality Schools.* A major way to find a good school for a child is for the family to move into a middle-class neighbor-hood with like-minded families, and well-supported, safe, and well-run schools. In fact, ask any local real estate agent, and he/she will tell a future buyer just how "excellent" the local schools are in the neighborhood—a major selling point for houses and apartments.

Even if prospective buyers do not have school-aged children, they will be interested in the reputation of the local schools, since resale demands and value of homes are often related to the perception of local school quality. This chapter will present the data on housing values and school quality, a first step in the interrelationship between school quality and family resources.

2. *Other Private School Options.* For families who prefer nonpublic schools for their children, the ability to "buy" a quality education pres-ents options that poorer families may not have. Thus, those with higher income have the options of enrolling their children in a local, regional, or even a national private (boarding) school. Currently, about 6 million chil-dren in the United States (out of 55 million total school children) attend a variety of private (nondenominational and religiously affiliated) K-12 schools.

A driving force for private and parochial schools may also be reli-gious, as 25 different religious groups (religions and sects) operate a range of schools that teach the secular subjects, and/or a particular religion, including Catholicism, Judaism, Protestantism, and Islam. And private schools may also be nonsectarian, such as military academies, Montessori schools, independent day and boarding schools, and programs with other themes such as music and art, dance, or foreign languages (e.g., French at a lycée).

3. *Extra Help.* Families with resources can also hire professionals to help their children learn a foreign language, to play a musical instrument, dance, and drama, or handle emotional, language/speech, and physical difficulties. In addition, parents of children needing extra academic and social assistance can have tutors, speech pathologists, psychologists, physical therapists, and others to help their children develop their talents, and deal with their difficulties and needs.

Also, students from more affluent and involved homes may experience greater intellectual, social, and artistic enrichment through travel, summer camps, museums, and various artistic and cultural events. Thus, the family can further reinforce the child's cultural and intellectual growth through access to books, online materials, and computer/technological equipment at home.

Families with these cultural and monetary-enriching resources can help their children at home, with homework and extracurricular activities, called "concerted cultivation" (authors), in addition to natural growth and development.

Private and Parochial Schools

Table 6.2 shows the private schools picture, with the total number of students in all private schools growing from 4.8 million in 1900 to 5.1 million enrolled by 2004. However, the most affordable private schools for poorer parents, the Catholic schools, have been seriously declining and continue to do so (Cattaro, 2002). In 1990, 11.4 percent of all school-age students went to private schools, of whom 48 percent were attending the nation's Catholic schools. But by 2002–2003, the percentage of total children in nonpublic schools remained fairly constant at 11.7 percent, while

Table 6.2   Trends in Private K-12 School Enrollments by Affiliations: 1989–1990 to 2003–2004 (Cooper and Baxter, 2009, p. 54)

School Year Ending	Total Private School Enrollment (in Thousands)	Roman Catholic %	Conservative Christian %	Affiliated %	Unaffiliated %	Nonsectarian %
1990	4,838	54.5	10.9	12.8	8.5	13.2
2004	5,123	46.2	15.1	10.8	9.9	18.0
Change	+ 285	- 8.3	+ 4.2	- 2.0	+ 1.4	+ 4.8

the Catholic percentage of private fell 9 percent to just 39 percent of the private sector, and only 4.6 percent of the total of school-age children in the United States. (Youniss and Convey, 2004).

Thus, Catholic schools that often served lower-income children (Buetow, 1970, 1983; Kraushaar, 1970), and now many ethnic groups (Latinos/as and African Americans) have been closing down at an alarming rate (see Lawrence, 2004), while private schools for more-affluent families, both independent and religious, have been increasing (Kraushaar, 1970). These changes are giving middle-class students more options, and poorer students less schools that they can afford. (Bryk, Lee, and Holland, 1993).

Figure 6.1 shows the Catholic school declines in those particular states with the largest Catholic enrollment; the drop has occurred in all major states except Florida, which has a large Latino/Latina population of immigrants, and has held constant in enrollments between the years 2000 and 2004 at around 93,000-plus students. (Cooper and D'Agustino, 2012).

Meanwhile, the large states, such as New York, Pennsylvania, Illinois, and Ohio witnessed the greatest declines, mainly because Catholic parish schools were closing in large cities such as New York City, Philadelphia, Chicago, and Cleveland, where the largest poor population lives—and perhaps the need for a Catholic school choice is greatest.

Thus, in the last 25 years, the largest and most inexpensive (thus affordable) private schools, those run in parishes and dioceses by the

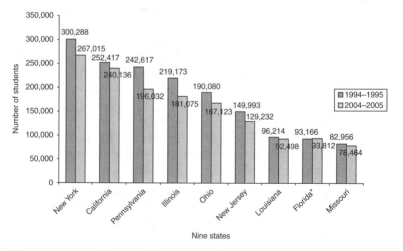

Figure 6.1   Data Showing Changes in Catholic School Enrollment by Largest Enrollment States, 1994–2004.

Source: Cooper, B. S. & D'Agustino, S. (2012). Catholic school survival and the common good: Trends, developments, and future directions. In Bauch (Ed). *Catholic schools in the public interest: Past, present and future trends* (pp. 156–167) Charlotte, NC: IAP.

Note: Florida enrollment numbers represent 1999/2000 as compared to 2004–2005

Roman Catholic church, have been declining and closing at an alarming rate. Every year, Catholic Archdioceses such as New York and Chicago have to close some 20 to 30 parish schools for lack of funds and leadership, as the number of nuns, priests, and brothers to help operate these schools has been shrinking (Cooper, 2008).

These schools have (had) much lower tuition (from about $1,900 to $2,300 per year), which enabled some less-affluent, upwardly mobile families—some of whom were not even Catholic themselves—to afford a private school for their children in the inner-city (Nelson, 2000).

Even charter schools, which often require that students' families make use of a lottery system, cannot serve the growing number of poorer children, and the chance of a poor kid gaining admission is based on chance (with few real chances) (see Weinberg, 2002). In fact, in the Archdiocese of Washington, DC—which has been closing Catholic schools at an alarming rate—the leader, Donald Cardinal Wuerl has been able to convert his failing, closing parish schools into publicly funded charter schools, as the Cardinal did not want to see the students pushed out on the street and forced to attend the failing, declining public schools. Now almost 40 percent of students in DC are attending charter schools, the highest percent for any school system in the United States, giving poor families the option as Catholic schools close.

And while the United States has expanded its precollege and college courses for the middle and upper classes, vocational and career training programs, have all but disappeared, in our high schools meaning that less academic, and poorer kids are given fewer options and face a difficult time completing high school with its academic rigor. Re-instituting career training in trades and vocations will raise graduation rates and guarantee a better opportunity of finding jobs and making a living.

National Results: Step-by-Step

We see three steps in the process: percentage of students attending K-12 schools, graduating, and going on to college and beyond—and its effects on their lives and income. Each step is important in giving better opportunities for a good job, higher income, better housing, and the improved chances of finding a good school for the next generation:

Step 1: Percent of Students Completing High School: According to the National Community Survey (2005), the national average, as of 2005, of people 25 and over who completed high school with a diploma is 86.3 percent, with three states at over 90 percent (Alaska the highest with 91.4 percent, and Minnesota and Wyoming tied for second place with 90.7 percent completion). The highest completing states appear, interestingly enough, to be more rural, western, and central states, which have low incoming immigrants and ethnics and people of color.

The lowest levels of high school graduates are Mississippi (77.3 percent) as the fifty-first ranking (the bottom) including the District of Columbia; Kentucky at 77.6 percent; and Texas at 78.1 percent. The major urban populated states are below the average, including New York ranked thirty-fourth (with 83.9 percent) and California with forty-third (80.4 percent).

2. Number and Percent Completing College: The next step is to see how much higher education is being completed in the United States with about 85 percent holding a high school diploma. Here the comparison is not state-by-state, since students often "go away" to college; but rather the United States is compared to other modern nations, to see how we have fared and have changed in our college graduation rates.

The College Board keeps tabs on college admissions and completion: it determined that Canada has the highest level of higher education attainment in the world, with 56 percent of it students earning at least an associates of arts degree, while the United States has only 40 percent getting higher education degrees. The situation is even worse for poorer and minority and non-English speaking families. As the College Board explains in an article in the *New York Times*:

> While almost 70 percent of high school graduates in the United States enroll in college within two years of graduating, only about 57 percent of students who enroll in a bachelor's degree program graduate within six years, and fewer than 25 percent of students who begin at a community college graduate with an associate's degree within three years. (Lewin, July 23, 2010, p. 1)

Lewin also explains:

> The problem is even worse for low-income students and minorities: only 30 percent of African-Americans ages 25–34, and less than 20 percent of Latinos in that age group, have an associate's degree or higher. And students from the highest income families are almost eight times as likely as those from the lowest income families to earn a bachelor's degree by age 24.

Effects of Education Attainment and Degrees

The next assumption that we discuss in this chapter is the effects of better and more education on starting salaries, family income, "lifetime earnings," and ultimately socioeconomic "class" standing. Children who finish and graduate from high school are going to get better jobs, earn more money, and presumably be enabled to get a good education for their children. Attending and then graduating from college boosts income (and lifetime earnings) even more, as Levin et al. (2007) have explained:

> Over a lifetime, higher earnings from a college degree reflect differences in starting salaries and in earning trajectories. Using CPS data from March 1998, 1999, and 2002, Jennifer Cheeseman Day and Eric C. Newburger estimate that, over a work life, individuals with a bachelor's degree working full time, year round, earn about one-third more than individuals who do not finish college and earn almost twice as much as individuals with a high school diploma. (p. 704)

And when groups are compared, based on the level of public investment in their education, we see disturbing results. As Levin et al. (2007) found:

> Across the U.S.A., the average shortfall is $900–1200 per year. Therefore, as an approximation, total public K-12 educational investment per black student is $20,000 less than per white student. Of course, this disparity is understated by the amount of further or compensatory expenditure that is needed to equalize educational outcomes of children from disadvantaged families. (p. 704)

Are Americans Staying In School Longer?

Along with the financial data, the report also shows that more Americans are staying in school longer than ever before. In 2000, 84 percent of American adults aged 25 and over had at least completed high school, and 26 percent continued to earn a bachelor's degree or higher, both all-time highs. But is this long enough? President Obama does not think so, since the world's students are attending schools longer and putting the United States at a disadvantage.

As President Obama (2009) commented:

> Now, I know longer school days and school years are not wildly popular ideas. Not with Malia and Sasha, not in my family, and probably not in yours. But the challenges of a new century demand more time in the classroom…Our school calendar is based upon the agrarian economy and not too many of our kids are working the fields today.

"Glass Ceiling" on Earnings Still Intact

While more education works in general in raising income, we do see limits to the "year of education/more income" ratio. A report by the US

Bureau of Labor Statistics states that while more American women than men have received bachelor's degrees every year since 1982, men with professional degrees may expect to cumulatively earn almost $2 million more than their female counterparts over their work lives.

Glass ceiling aside, however, Longley (2009) found that women who graduated from college do earn *about 76 percent more* than women with only a high school diplomas. Additional highlights from the report show:

- In 1999, average annual earnings ranged from $18,900 for high school dropouts to $25,900 for high school graduates, $45,400 for college graduates and $99,300 for the holders of professional degrees (medical doctors, dentists, veterinarians and lawyers).
- Over a work life, earnings for a worker with a bachelor's degree compared with one who had just a high school diploma increase by about $1 million for non-Hispanic Whites and about $700,000 for African Americans; Asians and Pacific Islanders; and Hispanics. Currently, almost 9-in-10 young adults graduate from high school and about 6-in-10 high school seniors go on to college the following year.

A separate report released in 1996, "What's It Worth? Field of Training and Economic Status: 1996," said among people with bachelor's degrees, those working full time in engineering earned the highest average monthly pay ($4,680), while those with education degrees earned the lowest ($2,802) in 1996. Thus, the more education individuals get, the more money they are likely to earn. And usually, those extra earnings are more than pocket change.

Data from the US Bureau of Labor Statistics indicate that median earnings increase at every level of education. In 2005, as Table 6.1 illustrates, people who finished high school earned almost $175 more every week compared with those who dropped out. People who completed an associate degree program netted more than $100 compared with high school graduates. How much is higher education worth in cold hard money? A college master's degree means $1.3 million more in lifetime earnings than a high school diploma, according to a recent report from the US Census Bureau.

The report entitled "The Big Payoff: Educational Attainment and Synthetic Estimates of Work-Life Earnings" (PDF) reveals that over an adult's working life, high school graduates can expect, on an average, to earn $1.2 million; those with a bachelor's degree, $2.1 million; and people with a master's degree, $2.5 million (Day and Newburger, 2002).

Persons with doctoral degrees earn an average of $3.4 million during their working lives, while those with professional degrees do best at $4.4 million.

"At most ages, more education equates with higher earnings, and the payoff is most notable at the highest educational levels," said Jennifer Cheeseman Day, coauthor of the report (see Day and Newburger, 2002). The figures are based on 1999 earnings projected over a typical work life, defined as the period from ages 25 through 64.

The Future Is Now

The United States stands at the crossroads: how to increase education quality *and* quantity, getting more students to graduate with higher standards and learning levels. The president of the University of Maryland university system, William E. Kirwin, sees the problems and suggests solutions: "We led the world in the 1980s, but we didn't build from there. If you look at people 60 and over, about 39–40 percent have college degrees, and if you look at young people, too, about 39–40 percent have college degrees. Meanwhile, other countries have passed us by."

And by not educating up the ladder from preschool to university, the nation faces the general economic problem of competing with growing nations such as China and Korea. Yet in some ways, the United States gives least time and support to workers, and thus we can be considered an "overworked society." Comparing the United States to other nations in the word, we see the following:

- At least 134 countries have laws setting the maximum length of the work week; the United States does not.
- In the United States, 85.8 percent of males and 66.5 percent of females work more than 40 hours per week. According to the International Labor Organization (ILO), "Americans work 137 more hours per year than Japanese workers, 260 more hours per year than British workers, and 499 more hours per year than French workers."
- American workers get less vacation time, since the US "remains the only industrialized country in the world that has no legally mandated annual leave nor does the US have a federal law requiring 'paid sick days'." So while US productivity has increased 400 percent, the workers are not benefiting from the profits. So education needs attention, and so do the employment, pay, and benefits too.

We know that collge education is costly, time-consuming, and demanding. Yet, in recent times, more youngsters are keen to get a college education. Wonder why? To know why college education is growing in demand, look at the benefits of going to college (see *Benefit.Of.net. Benefits of Going to College*, 2011).

1. *More Career Options* One of the most important reasons for anyone to attend college is the upper hand it gives with regards to jobs and career. A college graduate has a better chance of landing a job when compared to an individual with a high school qualification. Further, a college graduate also has better options and opportunities to progress in their career.

2. *Greater Monetary Benefits* A college graduate earns approximately one million dollars more as compared to a high school diploma. Graduates are paid better salaries for the same jobs as compared to lesser-educated individuals. Therefore, we should have less worries about the dollars spent on college education. Once students have completed the course, they will be more likely to earn back more than what they and their families have spent—being one of the major motivational factors that ensures people complete their college education.

3. *Insurance against Unemployment* Graduates are believed to have better and more job opportunities as compared to diploma holders. In the growing economy diploma holders and lesser-educated individuals are losing their jobs and their market. Even during phases of no work or less work opportunities, college graduates survive better in the job market. Their graduate degree holds them in good stead by providing job opportunities as per their skills. Thus, a college education provides more job security and thus helps to insure individuals against unemployment.

4. *Increased Marketability* A college education definitely increases individual's marketability in the job market. A bonus is added that gives graduates some preference as compared to diploma holders or lesser-qualified individuals. It not only increases chances of landing a job but also increases student's chances of being paid better for the same job.

5. *Better Standards of Living* Studies have shown that college education not only gives graduates a better job, but also healthier living. A college graduate is believed to have better health, exercise better, and smoke lesser. Call it the advantages of a college education or a rub-off of being in a better social set-up because of improved income and better job environment. Whatever the reasons, a college education definitely often means a better standards of living.

6. *Stronger Social Networking* College education is believed to lead to better social networking. Generally, college is not only a time when we study hard but also enjoy as much. Most of us never forget our college days or the fun we had with friends. In fact, some of our best buddies are those that we met in college. College is a time when we connect with several people because of our need to improve communication skills, because of the extra-curricular activities, and because of our need to establish contacts to pursue our dream careers. All this leads to a large network of friends and acquaintances that can really help us when we get into the real world to search for a job and to establish a career.

7. Improved Skills Last but not the least, a college education can improve *job* skills and also many *life* skills. In addition to gaining more knowledge on a subject of one's choice, the college environment provides opportunities for students to develop communication skills, social inter-action skills, analytical skills, and reasoning skills. These definitely go a long way in helping students establish and maintain social relationships when graduates go out into the real world.

Conclusion

We have seen in this chapter just how critical education is to the family and the nation. If the gap in education, between the United States and other nations, and within the country, continues we may have to face worse scenarios in the future. The National Center for Public Policy and Higher Education (2005) predicts:

> Personal income per capita in the United States is projected to decline from $21,591 in 2000 to $21,196 in 2020—a drop of $395 or 2% (in infla-tion-adjusted dollars). In contrast, according to the Bureau of Economic Analysis, personal income per capita had grown 41% nationally during the two decades prior to 2000. One consequence of such a decline in personal income would be a decrease in the nation's tax base.

However, in contrast, if states can narrow the gap between white and ethnic/racial groups, then our education system will improve, income will increase, and the United States will compete effectively in the world economy—again illustrating the interconnection between better education and a stronger, more equitable economy. And with high-tech methods, states, districts, and families can begin to track progress as *Education Week* (November 15, 2011) recently reported. Data, available and understandable, can help the student, the family, the schools, and the universities—to build the bridge to higher education in the future, as this Kentucky example explains:

Once Kentucky educators started sharing data about how high school students were doing after graduation, things started to change:

- University professors and high school teachers began comparing notes about their expectations in class. Rigor was ramped up.

- Transition courses were developed in high schools to help lagging students avoid remediation in college. Advanced placement restrictions were lifted to expose more students to college-level courses.
- The percentage of college-going students in Kentucky went up, and the need for remediation in college went down.

The resulting college- and career-readiness feedback reports are a tool for superintendents, principals, guidance counselors, school board members, college administrators, and parents to make decisions about education.

So, as the Kentucky case explains, better data for parents and professionals, showing students progress educational, can help the transition from high school to college. Again, the intersection of better education, along with potential income and better health care, to some degree depends on everyone knowing the score and tracking progress.

References

Bryk, A. S., Lee, V. E., & Holland, P. B. (1993). *Catholic schools and the common good.* Cambridge, MA: Harvard University Press.

Buetow, H. A. (1983). *A history of Catholic schools in the United States.* Washington, DC: National Catholic Education Association.

———. (1970). *Of singular benefit: The story of Catholic education in the U.S.* New York: Macmillan.

Cattaro, G. M. (2002). Immigration and pluralism in urban Catholic schools. *Education and Urban Society, 34*(2), 199–211.

Cidams, C. (2011). *Data driving college preparation.* November 15. Education Week. Retrieved from http://www.edweek.org/ew.

Cooper, B. S. (2008). Foreword, to *Religious charter schools: Legalities and practicalities,* by Lawrence D. Weinberg. Charlotte, NC: Information Age Publishing, iii–vii.

Cooper, B. S., & D'Agustino, S. (2012). Chapter 12—Catholic school survival and the common good: Trends, developments, and future directions. In P. Bauch (Ed.), *Catholic schools in the public interest: Past, present and future trends* (pp. 156–167). Charlotte, NC: Information Age Publishing.

Cooper, B. S., & Baxter, T. B. (2009). Private schools. In T. L. Good (Ed.), *21st Century education: A reference handbook,* vol. 2 (pp. 277–287). Thousand Oaks, CA: Sage Publications.

Day, J. C., & Newburger E. C. (2002), The big payoff: Educational attainment and synthetic estimates of work-life earnings. *Current Population Reports,* Washington, DC: US Censury Bureau (July, 2002).

Furstenberg, F. F. (2010, Spring). On a new schedule: Transitions to adulthood and family change. *Transitions to Adulthood. 20*(1), 43–51.

Juliet, J. (2011). *Benefits of going to college*. Retrieved from http://benefitof .netbenefits-of-going-to-college.

Kraushaar, O. F. (1970). *American nonpublic schools: Patterns in diversity*. Baltimore, MD: Johns Hopkins University Press.

Lawrence, S. (2004). "New" immigrants in the Catholic schools: A preliminary assessment. In J. Youniss & J. J. Convey (Eds.), *Catholic schools at the crossroads: Survival and transformation* (pp. 178–200). New York: Teachers College Press.

Levin, H. M., Belfield, C., Muennig, P., & Roused, C. (2007). The public returns to public educational investments in African-American males. *Economics Education Review, 26*, 700–709.

Lewin, T. (2010, July 23). Once a leader, the U. S. lags in college degrees. *New York Times*. Retrieved from www.nytimes.com/2010/07/23college.htm

Longley, R. (2009). Lifetime earnings soar with education. Retrieved from usgov-info.about.com/od/moneymatters/a/edandearnings.htm.

Mare, R. D. (1995). Changes in educational attainment and school enrollment. In Reynolds Farley (Ed.), *State of the Union: America in the 1990s*, vol. 1, Economic Trends (pp. 155–214). New York: Russell Sage Foundation.

McCarthy, A. (1983, April). Parochial schools: Still a focus for Catholic identity. *Commonwealth*. April 1983, 232–233.

McCloskey, N. J. (1969). *Catholic education faces its future*. Garden City, NY: Double Day.

National Center for Public Policy and Higher Education (2005, November). IMPROVE Income of U.S. work force projected to decline if education doesn't improve. *Policy Alert*. San Jose, CA: The author.

National Community Survey (2005).*Percent of people who have completed high school (including equivalency) most recent by state*. Retrieved from www .statemaster.com/

Nelson, M. S. (2000). Black Catholic schools in inner-city Chicago: Forging a path to the future. In James Youniss & John J. Convey (Eds.), *Catholic schools at the crossroads: Survival and transformation* (pp. 157–177). New York: Teachers College Press.

———. (1998). Catholic elementary schools in Chicago's black inner city: Four modes of adaptation to environmental changes. *Nonprofit and Voluntary Sector Quarterly, 23*(3), 209–225.

Obama, B. (2009, August 1). School is out but education doesn't end for Obama daughters. *New York Times*. Retrieved from www.nytimes.com/2009/08/02/ summerhtm

Romboy, D. (2000, July 11). Human capital called key to U.S. success in Information Age. *Deseret New,* D6 & D8.

US Bureau of Labor Statistics (2005).*The big payoff: Educational Attainment and synthetic estimates of work-life earnings*. PDF file.

Weinberg, L. (2002). *The Constitutionality of Religion-based Charter Schools: Answering the Practical Legal Questions (2004)*. Dissertation completed at Boston University, College of Education.

Youniss, J., & Convey, J. J. (Eds.) (2004). *Catholic schools at the crossroads: Survival and transformation*. New York: Teachers College Press.

7

Adult Education Everywhere for Everyone

Introduction: Origins of the Problem

Adults with little or no formal education often confront problems since their opportunities to earn a decent living in a modern, competitive, hi-tech society are often challenged. How does a person grow up and receive relatively little/less education? What effects, for example, does not receiving a high school diploma have on an adult's life-chances, health, and annual income (Gould and Edward, 2011)?

And what can a modern society do to ensure that no individual reaches adulthood without a good education and adequate training, so women and men can find good jobs, earn descent livings, be healthy, and prosperous? And importantly, therefore, what can be done to provide education for people over age 20 who are not already graduated from high school, and even college, helping them to be better prepared for jobs and life?

Murray (1989) explains the difficulties of interpreting the data on why some grown-ups are impoverished in our society. He uses a metaphor, "Poverty is the elephant of social policy, with social scientists playing the role of the groping blind men [and women]" (p. 989). Murray then points out that a typical poor adult is impoverished for a set of different, complex reasons, while other similar adults are sometimes doing better economically.

And the most recent data on family income, poverty, and costs show that almost half of American families, even those with working parents, are living at what is barely seen as "adequate" (Cooper, 2011). As Table 7.1 shows, the 2009 poverty level for a one-person household was about $11,000 and went up about $4,000 for each other member from 2 in the household to around $37,000 for an eight-member family.

Table 7.1   2009 Poverty Guidelines: US Department of Health and Human Services

Persons in Family or Household	US Dollars
1	$10,830
2	14,570
3	18,310
4	22,050
5	25,790
6	29,530
7	33,270
8	37,010
For each additional person, add	3,740

Source: Information Courtesy of the National Center for Children in Poverty (www.nccp.org)

Four Important Questions About Child Poverty and Family Economic Hardship

Furthermore, we have seen an enormous growth in the number of people with incomes from 1.0 to 1.99 times the poverty threshold. This means that the number of Americans with incomes at or below 200 percent of the poverty line—a level often thought of as an adequate, but modest standard of living—has risen from 34 percent under the official measure to 47.5 percent under the "social policy model" (SPM). That's nearly half of all Americans.

Data are collected on "net worth" of families, finding that in general older people are more likely to own their homes and car plus other goods. As one study explained (*Education Week,* November 11, 2011, p. 1):

> Net worth includes the value of a person's home, possessions and savings accumulated over the years, including stocks, bank accounts, real estate, cars, boats or other property, minus any debt such as mortgages, college loans and credit card bills. Older Americans tend to hold more net worth because they are more likely to have paid off their mortgages and built up more savings from salary, stocks and other investments over time. The median is the midpoint, and thus refers to a typical household. (*Education Week,* November 7, 2011, p. 1)

This chapter assumes that many people have reached adulthood with a useful, complete education that helps them—people of age 18 or older—to do well in the health/education/welfare intersection. In particular, we focus on those who are for various reasons, not well-educated—and examine what leaders of society can do to provide these adults with a good and useful education, or renew the ones that have education and degrees—given that they often passed through K-12 schools without learning and practicing the skills they needed (Cambron-McCabe, 1993). We are seeking to learn about four critical realities about why some adults are poorly prepared and educated—and what can be done to help them:

1) Why do adults need further education in their lives, based on the absence of an adequate education when younger, and the changing demands of society?
2) Why are certain groups of adults unable to receive an adequate education in their younger lives, moving into adulthood?
3) What effects does being a poorly educated adult have on family income and opportunities to earn a good living and enjoy a healthy life?
4) What have societies, such as the United States and Europe, done to help adults keep up in the fields, work, and moving into the future, including military education and training?

Nature of the Problem

Adults, who were unable or unwilling to get a good education in their younger days, fall into several categories:

- Being poor without family stability and without consistent access to formal elementary-high school and then college education;
- Being a recent immigrant from a less-developed country where a full education may not have been available, and thus young people moved to the United States ill-prepared for school and learning (in English);
- Being a school dropout or "push-out" during youth when schooling became difficult and inconsistent;
- Being incarcerated for breaking the law, which interrupts and weakens education progress and the learning of basic skills;
- Being abused and neglected as a child, and/or;
- Being children with special problems and needs who were unable to get and pass through the basic stages of learning in K-12 schools.

All these conditions and situations are more common than readily apparent, and may cause individuals to grow into and pass through adulthood without completing elementary, middle, and/or high school. Many young people do not make it into college and/or gain college degrees and diplomas to prepare them for work and life. These students may have limited opportunities to learn a skill, or a trade.

Thus, entering a high-paying professional field is unlikely; and these adults may find it difficult to find profitable employment in a trade, skill area, profession, or service job, although many jobs do exist for adults without the traditional university-graduate/professional school education.

Several national and international data studies have been done, comparing adult literacy and numeracy between 1992 and 2003 in the United States by ethnicity and background of adults, and then showing these comparative data in several other nations. The Adult Literacy and Life-Skills (ALL) data were gathered and compared by group, and found, for example, that

> in 1992 and 2003, White and Asian/Pacific Islander adults had higher average scores than their Black and Hispanic peers in the three types of literacy assessed. Black performance increased in each type of literacy from 1992 to 2003, while Hispanic average scores declined in prose and document literacy. (US Department of Education, 2007)

Additional differences in average literacy were thus apparent by education and age. Educational attainment is positively related to all three types of literacy: those with any education after high school outperformed their peers with less education in 1992 through 2003. Between these years, average prose literacy decreased for adults at most levels of educational attainment, and average document literacy decreased for those with some college, associate's degrees, and college graduates. From 1992 to 2003, the average prose (related to reading and writing), document (related to social studies and some sciences), and quantitative literacy (math and most sciences) scores of adults aged 50–64 and 65 or older increased.

Recognition of "adult education problems" can be traced back to the Enlightenment and great thinkers such as Rousseau (1772) who advised the Polish government that "it is education that must give souls a national formation, and direct their opinions and tastes in such a way that they will be patriotic by inclination, passion, by necessity" (p. 22). Thus, besides education—and the lack of it—affecting the individual and family, such learning also has major effects on the nation, the society, and the overall quality of life in a nation.

We know, as Malcolm Tight (2000) explains, that adult learning should and does go on over a lifetime:

> Adult education and training—now widely re-labeled and re-energize under the banner of *lifelong learning*—are an important and developing field of activity and study. We are all, as children and adults, engaged in learning every day of our lives... We are all increasingly likely to be

involved in more formalized forms of learning and training—both immediately after we have completed [or dropped out of] the compulsory education period and throughout our lives. (p. 1)

While these programs and education services are sometimes available
to adults throughout their lives, we know that they are neither equitable
nor effective for all. These problems of access and effectiveness are not
simply common in the United States. We see in Europe, for example, a
recognition that

> participation in adult education remains highly unequal. Those most
> in need participate the least. Finding new ways to motivate and involve
> excluded groups is a high priority for policy, research and funding. This
> requires a shift from supply- to demand-driven policy, a focus on diver-
> sity of provision to meet different individuals' and group needs, and more
> support for locally determined adult learning opportunities. (European
> Association for the Education of Adults, 2006, p. 26)

In the United States, poor cities such as Detroit have some of the highest
levels of adult functional illiteracy, including those with a high schools
diploma, in the nation. As one report explained:

> According to estimates by The National Institute for Literacy, roughly
> 47 percent of adults in Detroit, Michigan—200,000 total—are "function-
> ally illiterate," meaning they have trouble with reading, speaking, writing
> and computational skills. Even more surprisingly, the Detroit Regional
> Workforce finds half of that illiterate population has obtained a high
> school degree. (*Huffington Post*, November 12, 2011)

Educating Adults, Where and When?

Given the importance of education for adults, for those unable or unwilling to get a solid education in the youth and childhood, our society has a
wide range and variety of programs to extend an opportunity to adults to
catch up and learn new skills—while also polishing their old ones.

Thus, adult education is available virtually everywhere: for example,
a range of graduate programs, in-service and professional development,
adult training classes, high school, and trade school certificates. Yet,
rarely have government officials or education specialists taken a system-
atic look at the following: (1) What types and how much adult education
programs are needed and are now available in each region of the country? (2) What needs and demands exist for these programs across groups,
fields, levels, and skill area? (3) How many and which adults take part in
these training efforts, whether at their business or at regional colleges and

center? And (4) based on their availability, what are the net results from this training in terms of:

(a) Increased mobility and access to jobs,

(b) Real income growth based on more preparation and better jobs with the current industry of site, and by moving to new jobs with better pay and benefits, and,

(c) Future needs for adult education in changing economies and fields.

Formal Adult Education

The traditional forms of education begin with higher and extended education that starts in college and university, into professional and graduate schools and periodically throughout life. Every community has some range and types of adult education programs that can be categorized as *Liberal-Classical Tradition, Behaviorists, Progressive, and Humanistic.* Each type of adult education has a different philosophy-purpose, learner, and teacher.

For example, a number of schools, such as Penn Foster in Scranton, PA, are the largest accredited adult education school for independent study. It offers courses online, making it the largest distance-learning institution in the world, as the mission statement explains: "The school provides programs and services that are designed to meet the lifelong learning needs of the adult learner, leading to career-specific diplomas" (www.pennfoster.edu/about_us.html). So, adults who want and need the education can take a distance-learning program, working for diplomas that qualify them for job and careers.

So adults already employed could take courses and prepare themselves for promotion; or people looking for a job might be boosted up the application list, get interviewed, and increase the chances of landing a job. The list of online courses is staggering, from high school level to college, technician and accounting, for licensing and accrediting. So adult education is out there, and is complex, and has been observed and evaluated by the US Department of Education. The National Center for Education Statistics has been collecting data on adult education and progress for years, and been evaluating the results, as explained:

A wide variety of evaluation projects have been funded under Adult Education National Programs since beginning in FY 1988. The Office of Vocational and Adult Education (OVAE), the Office of the Under Secretary, Planning and Evaluation Service (OUS), or the Office of Educational Research and Improvement (OERI) have administered these projects. The projects funded have ranged from small commissioned papers to large-scale nationally representative surveys and a random assignment experiment of a welfare reform program involving adult education. New studies are focusing on assessment of the impact of programs for special target populations and development of models of effective programs. (Silverberg, Warner, Fong, and Goodwin, 2004)

The department sought to determine, among other results, (1) How well the programs used technology to improve direct instruction and

Table 7.2   Adult Education: Purpose, Learner, and Teacher

	Liberal (Classical, Traditional)	Behaviorist, Practical	Progressive	Humanistic	Radical
Purpose	To develop intellectual powers of the mind; to make a person literate in the broadest sense—intellectually, morally, and spiritually.	To bring about behavior that will ensure survival of human species, societies, and individuals; to promote behavioral change.	To transmit culture and societal structure to promote social change; to give learner practical knowledge and problem-solving skills; to reform society.	To develop people open to change and continued learning; to enhance personal growth and development; to facilitate self-actualization, to reform society.	To bring about fundamental, social, political, and economic changes in society through education; to change culture and its structure.
Learner	"Renaissance person"; cultured, always a learner; seeks knowledge rather than just information; conceptual; theoretical understanding.	Learner plays an active role in learning, practicing new behavior, and receiving feedback; strong environmental influence.	Learner needs, interests, and experiences are key elements in learning; people have unlimited potential to be developed through education.	Learner is highly motivated and self-directed; assumes responsibility for learning and self-development.	Equality with teacher in learning process; personal autonomy; people create history and culture by combining reflection with action.
Teacher	The "expert"; transmitter of knowledge; authoritative; clearly directs learning process.	Manager; controller; predicts and directs learning outcomes; designs learning environment that elicits desired behavior.			

administration? (2) How adult education affected welfare reform locally and statewide? and (3) How adult education helped to improve local and state performance and evaluation outcome data?

Table 7.2 presents four common notions of adult education, including liberal (classical-traditional), behaviorist-practical, progressive, humanistic, and radical, with their purposes, types of learner, and role of the teacher.

Now that we have discussed the types of adult education—and the importance of it to families and society—we now look at some real examples including adult education in the military, in vocational and technical programs in colleges or run by industry, and other locations.

Military Training

The US military has long been a source of education for adult who are drafted and/or who enlist in the air forces: for example, navy, marines, air forces, and army. This training starts in a boot camp (basic training) and continues through specialization and increases with promotion into the officer corps. For the elites who are nominated by their senators and get accepted to attend Annapolis (naval academy), West Point (army), and air force and coast guard academies, education is explicitly leading to a bachelors of science, adult education is part of the program. But for those who are enlisted, the skills that may be learned are more basic, and can be useful in finding employment after leaving the armed forces.

Others can combine their military training with their college work, as the advertisement from Armed Forces Education (AFE) explains:

> Let us help you find military friendly colleges and discover your military college benefits. As a higher education portal, we're dedicated to helping you explore degree programs at military colleges. And when it's time to pay for your education, we're committed to offering information on military college benefits so you better understand your options. (Military.com. education.training)

At the start, as with all adult education, the military program includes learning the basic math and literacy skills, with the military program (Army Regulation 621–5) called *Functional Academic Skills Training (FAST)*. The military also helps students finish school and attend college, as this advertisement explains:

> The military has taught you how to succeed, giving you the experience that employers are looking for. Now, you just need to earn your degree.

Let ArmedForcesEDU.com connect you with military-friendly schools, to "service-members opportunity colleges" and make sure you're on the path to accomplishing your goals. (Military.com.education.training)

Here are some key areas of military education for adults:

1. **Education Benefits to Active Adults in the Military:** Current military members can use Military Tuition Assistance to pay for their education. Tuition Assistance, TA, offers $250 per semester credit hour for eligible military students.
2. **Benefits for Veterans:** Eligible veterans can apply for the Post 9/11 GI Bill or the Montgomery GI Bill, with Post 9/11 also an option of using the Yellow Ribbon Program to cover unpaid education expenses.
3. **Educational Benefits for Spouses:** Eligible spouses can apply for MyCAA, Military Spouse Career Advancement Accounts—a program for spouses pursuing an education.
4. **Additions to the Military Tuition Assistance for College:** An Active Duty military member can use Tuition Assistance, with Top-up to cover any remaining tuition costs. As part of the Montgomery GI Bill-Active Duty program, the VA pays the Top-up Benefit.
5. **First Step for the GI Bill?** First is the Veterans ON-line APPlication (VONAPP) website, including VA Form 22–1990, Application for Education Benefits.
6. **Cover All College Education Costs:** As of August 1, 2011, the Yellow Ribbon Program will pay out-of-state tuition at a public school. The program is also available to attend a private or foreign school when tuition and fees exceed $17,500 per year. With the Yellow Ribbon Program, the college agrees to pay a portion of the remaining tuition and fees and the VA matches that portion and issues payment directly to the institution.
7. **Level of Funding with the Post 9/11 GI Bill In- and Out-of-State:** With the Post 9/11 GI Bill, the GI Bill amount will cover all in-state tuition and fees at degree-granting public schools and will pay the different in out-of-state schools under the Yellow Ribbon Program. If you attend an out-of-state public school, you will receive the cost of in-state tuition at that school and can use the Yellow Ribbon Program to pay for the rest, as long as the school participates in the Yellow Ribbon Program.

As of October 1, 2011, Post 9/11 GI Bill will pay tuition for nondegree programs, such as vocational or certificate programs. The Post 9/11

GI Bill pays the actual cost for in-state tuition at the school or $17,500, whichever is less.

8. **Payment under the Montgomery GI Bill:** The funding depends on the current full-time monthly entitlement amount. After two years of honorable service, prorated portion of the funds are available; and after three years, 100 percent of the funds are given.
9. **Payment of Loans for Deployed Military:** Payment on college loans begins after being away from classes for 29 days.
10. **College Credit for Military Training:** Each armed service provides transfer credit to college for military training with the consent of the colleges: Navy/Marines visit the SMART website. Army visit the AARTS website. And Air Force visit the CCAF website. On each website, you can learn how your military training transfers to college courses. Then, check with the college you wish to attend to determine what training will transfer to college credit there.
11. **College Education for Disabilities through the Vocational Rehabilitation and Employment Program:** The program helps those with service-connected disabilities receive educational and vocational training.

Thus, adult can learn much from the military programs, as a means for advancing higher education for adults with service in the military. The most famous is the GI Bill, which takes veterans and gives them a second chance at higher education at reduced costs, tuition funds to attend college to earn a higher education degree.

Vocational-Technical Education

Another model of adult education is training to work as technicians in industry and governments. Named after Representative Carl D. Perkins, onetime Congressman from Kentucky, and major supporter of vocational education for adults and teenagers, we see the government making the connection between a good, practical education and better pay and benefits:

The Office of Vocational and Adult Education (OVAE), Division of Academic and Technical Education (DATE), administers the Carl D. Perkins Career and Technical Education Act (Perkins) and is responsible for helping all students acquire challenging academic and technical skills and be prepared for high-skill, high-wage, or high-demand occupations in the 21st century global economy. (The Office of Vocational and Adult Education [OVAE])

These technical training initiatives are provided in different ways by the three layers of government: (1) a federal role in running discretionary and formula-driven national programs for teaching adults technology and crafts; (2) support from state offices to offer discretionary programs, to improve programs, implementation, and accountability/assessment; And (3) local training programs that are available, rigorous, and accountable (Cambron-McCabe, 2002).

Table 7.3 shows the level of participation in vocation-occupations programs, and the credit that can be earned using 2005 national data.

As we see in Table 7.3, a range of occupations and skill areas are covered in these adult programs, with the majority majoring in a broad category ("any occupational area"), and "business," "communications," "agriculture," and "computers" coming next.

Yet another way to look at national data is to determine the link between high school study and continuing and adult education, by field. Table 7.4 presents percentages of adult study begun in high school and continued and completed after high school

We see the connections, then, in practical terms, for what adults study post-high schools, compared to what they were studying in high school. So the roots of vocational and technical, professional, and business training often begin during adolescence, as students realize that what they were studying in high school was applicable to their lives and training postsecondary and into adulthood.

Perhaps the groups of adults with the greatest difficulty to find employment are those that are of working age, but are "unemployed," about 9 percent of the nation in 2011. And current news is not good, from the Bureau of Labor Statistics (November 2, 2011):

> Last Friday's Job Openings and Labor Turnover data release from the Bureau of Labor Statistics offered further proof that there are not enough jobs for the nation's unemployed workers. With a meager increase of 225,000 job openings in September, the latest job openings numbers did little to reduce the imbalance between job openings and unemployment. At 4.2-to-1, September job-seeker's ratio (the ratio of unemployed to job openings) means that for more than three out of four unemployed workers, there are no jobs to be found. (Economic Policy Institute, 2011, p. 1)

Thus, to have a better education and be a prepared adult community will neither create nor mean easy, available jobs if the jobs don't exist. Thus, the economic condition of the nation, related to employment opportunities, will mean fewer workers on the job, and thus less income and benefit (health and welfare).

Table 7.3 Percentage of Public High School Graduates Who Concentrated in Each Occupational Area, by Number of Occupational Credits Earned, 2005

Occupational Concentration	2-Credit Occupational Concentrators[1]			3-Credit Occupational Concentrators[2]		
	All Graduates (%)	Graduates Who Earned Any Occupational Credits (%)	Graduates Who Earned 2.0 or More Occupational Credits (%)	All Graduates (%)	Graduates Who Earned Any Occupational Credits (%)	Graduates Who Earned 3.0 or More Occupational Credits (%)
Any occupational concentration	33.8	44.7	68.6	21.3	24.5	54.1
Agriculture and natural resources	4.7	5.5	8.4	2.9	3.4	7.5
Business	8.5	9.7	15.0	3.1	3.5	7.8
Communications and design	5.4	6.2	9.5	2.0	2.4	5.2
Computer and information sciences	3.7	4.3	6.5	1.4	1.6	3.6
Construction and architecture	2.1	2.5	3.8	1.2	1.4	3.1
Consumer and culinary services	4.4	5.0	7.7	2.2	2.5	5.6
Engineering technologies	2.4	2.8	4.3	1.0	1.2	2.6
Health sciences	3.2	3.7	5.7	2.1	2.5	5.4
Manufacturing, repair, and transportation	7.5	8.6	13.3	4.5	5.2	11.5
Marketing	2.6	3.1	4.7	1.4	1.6	3.6
Public services	1.2	1.4	2.1	0.6	0.7	1.5

Source: US Department of Education, Institute of Education Sciences, National Center for Education Statistics, High School Transcript Study (HSTS), 2005.

Notes
[1] 2-credit occupational concentrators are defined as graduates who earned 2.0 or more credits in any one of the 11 occupational areas listed in this table.
[2] 3-credit occupational concentrators are defined as graduates who earned 3.0 or more credits in any one of the 11 occupational areas listed in this table.

This table shows, for example, that among all public high school graduates from the class of 2005, 4.7 percent completed a 2-credit occupational concentration in agriculture and natural resources. Also, 5.5 percent of graduates who earned any occupational credits completed a 2-credit occupational concentration in agriculture and natural resources. The total weighted count of public high school graduates in 2005 was 2.4 million. Detail may not sum to totals because of rounding.

Table 7.4   Relationship between High School and Postsecondary Fields of Study in 2006 Compared to 2004 Secondary School Students

Area of Concentration[1]	Percentage	95% Confidence Interval
2-credit occupational concentrators	**18.1**	[15.4–20.7]
Agriculture and natural resources	**12.5**	[6.3–18.7]
Business	**24.1**	[18.8–29.4]
Communications and design	**12.6**	[7.8–17.3]
Computer and information sciences	**13.5**	[7.5–19.6]
Construction and architecture	**14.2**	[3.2–25.1]
Consumer and culinary services	**7.9**	[1.8–14.1]
Engineering technologies	**11.8**	[4.1–19.5]
Health sciences	**32.8**	[23.1–42.4]
Manufacturing	#	[†]
Marketing	**5.1**	[1.3–9.0]
Public services	**17.7**	[0.9–34.5]
Repair and transportation	**18.2**	[8.6–27.9]
3-credit occupational concentrators	**18.7**	[15.0–22.3]
Agriculture and natural resources	**15.4**	[6.9–24.0]
Business	**26.1**	[16.8–35.3]
Communications and design	**16.5**	[7.8–25.2]
Computer and information sciences	**18.1**	[4.6–31.6]
Construction and architecture	‡	[†]
Consumer and culinary services	**12.4**	[1.1–23.8]
Engineering technologies	**12.1**	[0.0–25.2]
Health sciences	**30.8**	[18.4–43.2]
Manufacturing	#	[†]
Marketing	**9.3**	[0.9–17.7]
Public services	‡	[†]
Repair and transportation	**24.3**	[8.6–40.0]

Source: US Department of Education, National Center for Education Statistics, Education Longitudinal Study of 2002 (ELS:2002), "Second Follow-up, 2006" and High School Transcript Study (HSTS), 2004.

Notes:
[†] Not applicable.
Rounds to zero.
‡ Reporting standards not met.
[1] The 2- and 3-credit occupational concentrators are graduates who earned at least 2.0 and 3.0 credits, respectively, in one of the 12 occupational areas listed in the table. Graduates can concentrate in more than one occupational area.

Evaluating Adult Education in America

The field of adult education is large and complex, reflecting the diversity of the types of work available to grown-ups at different levels and with interests in the market. While traditional high school education is primarily subject-centered (e.g., math, science, and social studies), adult education is much more focused and practical, centered on skills (e.g., welding and repairing) and areas (communications and health sciences) and levels (from high school through higher education and vocational education).

This section presents some models used to evaluate the quality and effects of adult education, based on a book by Thomas R. Guskey (2000), *Evaluating Professional Development*. Guskey explains ways and steps to evaluate and improve adult education, using the "staff development" model. Key to this approach is the work of Donald L. Kirkpatrick (1994), who has conceptualized the training evaluation development model in four (and later five) steps consisting of

1) **Reaction:** how the learners react to the learning process
2) **Learning:** the extent to which the learners gain knowledge and skills
3) **Behavior:** capability to perform the learned skills while on the job
4) **Results:** includes such items as monetary, efficiency, moral, and so on
5) **Responding to New Needs:** includes updating training as industry, commerce, and services change.

Note that the *Behavior* step involves job-skills and that the final outcomes, the *results*, include items such as money (salary), efficiency, moral, and other benefits. These outcomes are different from K-12 student outcomes where job skills and salary are obviously never assessed for children.

Level 1: Reaction: Guskey (2000) summarizes the first step in the Kirkpatrick method, states that we need to know "how participants regard their job development experience, whatever form it takes…their reactions to a formal presentation, workshop, course, seminar, or institute" (2000, p. 94). This first step is regarded as the easiest to assess, the directly related to the "how" of the adult education program. And they focus on the knowledge, skills, and practices of the lesson. Adult education, to help participants to prepare or advance in their work and careers, is direct and immediate.

And the questions are very practical, as Guskey explains, focusing on the facilities, room size, and equipment, and so are other "accommodations" appropriate for the activities—even the room is at the right temperature and well-lit, chair are comfortable, refreshments are fresh, tasty, and adequate. Adults have stronger opinions on food and lighting than most children in school. Oral questions, questionnaires, and levels of expectations and fulfillment characterize evaluations of adult education programs, whether in a college, community center, or in on-the-job programs.

Level 2: Participants' Learning: Adult education, at whatever level and for whatever purpose, works to teach, and is evaluated by seeing what students (adults) have actually learned, what skills they've built, and even their beliefs and attitude. Guskey (2000) puts it quite up front when he writes that changes may "stem from, for example, involvement in workshops, courses, seminars, institutes, curriculum development projects, study group experiences, or action research" (p. 121), where students do practical activities around their interests and programs. Thus, goals can be cognitive, psychomotor, affective (emotional), academic, skill development, and attitudinal.

Level 3: Participant's Behavior: Professional development programs are instituted to groups of adult learners to improve understanding of theory and implementation of activities within the school environment. The Behavior evaluation, according to Guskey (2000), "is the extent to which the trainees applied the learning and changed their behavior" (p. 7). The issue at hand might be how these changes in behavior are evaluated and measured to ensure improvement in application. Thus a system of assessment should be both supportive, positive and ongoing.

Level 4: Results evaluation measures the effect on the school, classroom or environment. The use of data either in performance or other goal-oriented activities assesses the return on the training and skill implementation. According to the plan and expected outcome, the assessments can be cognitive, academic, skill based and/or affective. Thus clear expectations must be in place before results can be measured and evaluated. Using a results plan can be affective when the participants understand the goals and expectations during or at the completion of a class or lesson.

Level 5: Responding to New Needs: Responding to New Needs: Guskey (2000) explains, "What was the impact on students? Did the professional development program or activity benefit students in any way" (p. 8). The information based on assessment can lead to new improvements, adjustments and/or new strategies for future training and program changes.

Planning the Future

This chapter has shown the needs for adults, their learning and skill-building, and the resources available to them (Massarella, 1980). The nation needs to continue on the road to literacy, numeracy, and skills development, which should help employment, raise and sustain family income, and thus increase the resources to buy better health care and nutrition. But we need data on the following key variables:

1. **Adults, by Age and Education:** We need to know how many adults are educated and to what levels. If researchers started with local public schools, what we know about their students over the last decade: how many enrolled, what their averages and credit accumulation were, and how many graduated or didn't from high school and beyond.

2. **Non-High School Graduates:** We then could take a cohort of adults who did not officially finish high school, and see what jobs, further education, and incomes they had earned. Case studies of these adults would be interesting, to see how they may have accumulated credits, graduated high school, and moved on to further to higher education—and what effects this preparation had on on-the-job opportunities and income.

3. **Military Men and Women:** We know that a percentage of adults enter the armed services, serve their country, and usually return to civilian life. What effects and results were gained from military service, promotions, and retirement that can then be related to the men and women's occupations, work, income, and health-care access? We also know that a small but significant percentage of young adults enter the "officer corps," usually by attending a military academy or enlisting in the Reserve Officers Training Corps (ROTC) in college/university. They graduate with a BA or BS, and are placed into the officers' ranks and serve their country in the active military for three to four years, or more?

Some nations, such as Israel, require all able young adults—men and women—to join and serve in military for four years, before entering college or going to work. This model may be an equalizer and provide young people with a chance to be treated as mature people between ages 17 and 23. We need to know where these adults are in the United States, what further education and training they receive, and what degrees and certificates they may earn.

4. **Looking Forward:** Finally, US leaders, educators, employers, service providers, all need to meet and see where we stand. Can we predict what jobs and opportunities are "out there" and forthcoming? What degrees and skills will these adults need in the future? What agencies and schools/universities are able and willing—and can afford—to provide opportunities for adults to

learn new skills, and how industry can continue to upgrade the knowledge and preparation of its employees for the next ten years or more? (Zinn, 1990).

We already know that online education is working, beaming courses into homes, schools, and business, to help everyone learn and keep up. Government at the federal, state, and local levels needs to support and expand these learning opportunities. Students while in K-12 schools should get a chance to use the latest technology, a modern model of the earlier voc-tech education that still exist is some regions and cities. For example, Automotive High School in New York City teaches high school students to tune and repair cars, from the outside in: bodywork, painting, repairs, engine workings, and fixings the interior of the vehicle (Louis and Miles, 1990).

These students (and other adults in the field) should be exposed to the latest high-tech electronic propulsion models, since the future is coming as cars and trucks continue to develop from diesel and gas-driven to electronic, and sun power. Keeping up, catching up, and looking ahead go hand in hand.

The whole process, from planning to evaluating, can help improve the education of adults at various stages: high school, college, military, work, and even in prison. Guskey (2000) understood the importance of knowing and evaluating the programs, when he wrote:

> Evaluation is an evolving, ongoing process, not a one-time event with a clear beginning and definite end. Evaluation purposes change through planning, formative and summative evaluation stages. Evaluation methods also change in response to the *level of evaluation,* ongoing refinements in programs and activities, and an alteration in stakeholders' needs. (p. 273)

This evaluation model also applies to the planning and implementation stages, as our society works to educate, prepare, employ, and promote adults in a complex social and economic environment (D. Sparks, 1994, G. M. Sparks, 1983). For we need to prepare and support a whole new generation of educators, as Guskey explains: "It is increasingly important to prepare a generation of teachers and school administrators who see themselves as advocates for low-income communities rather than paternalistic leaders with a deficit model of urban children and their parents" (2000, p. 305).

Thus, not only is adult education for the poor, undereducated dropouts, but it is also for the educational professionals (principal, superintendents, and teachers), who are critical adults themselves. These educators are learning to help younger students and adults to be well-prepared, so that they and their families can make a real living, get good health care, and see that their children. Thus the next generation can receive a good education as children and adults (in college, the military, at work, and online). Some call this "social justice," while others simply refer to it as good education for all. Collaboration is essential, as Adler and Gardner (1994) relate these groups and levels:

The child

- *to the family (primary caregivers),*
- *to schools, social services, health care, and recreation,*
- *to government agencies/foundations/universities,*
- *to funding, regulations, and training providers,*
- *to political forces (unions, profession associations, special interest groups) and finally*
- *to the whole society.*

Thus, intersecting *horizontally* across health, education, and welfare also requires a *vertical* relationship among the child, family, community, schools, and society. These conditions work in both direction, to help children and adults to learn and do better today and into the future.

References

Adler, L., & Gardner, S. (Eds.) (1994). *The politics of linking schools and social services.* New York: Taylor & Francis, LLC.

Cambron-McCabe, N. (2002). Educational accountability in the USA: Focus on state testing. *Education and the Law, 14*(1), 117–126.

———. (1993). Leadership for democratic authority. In J. Murphy (Ed.), *Preparing tomorrow's school leaders: Alternative designs.* University Park, PA: UCEA.

Cooper, P. (2011, November 9). "Working economics": Census tries to better identify poverty and finds what? More of it. See blog of the Economic Policy Institute.

Education Week (November 7, 2011). U.S. Wealth Gap Between Young and Old Is Widest Ever. New York: Associated Press, p. 1.

European Association for the Education of Adults (2006). *Adult education trends and issues in Europe.* Brussels, Belgium: Author.

Gould, E., & Edwards, K. A. (2011). Another look at poverty in the Great Recession. *Research Ideas for Shared Prosperity.* Washington, DC: Economic Policy Institute.

Guskey, T. R. (2000). *Evaluating professional development.* Thousand Oaks, CA: Corwin-Sage Publications.

Huff Post Business (2011, November 12) *Huffington Post*, 1.

Holloway, L. (2011). Government aid helped cut poverty rate. Retrieved from www.theroot.com/buzz/november12

Kirkpatrick, D. L. (1994). Evaluating training programs: Evidence vs. proof. *Training and Development Journal, 31*(11), 9–12.

Louis, K. S., & Miles, M. B. (1990). *Improving the urban high school: What works and why.* New York: Teachers College Press.

Massarella, J. A. (1980). Synthesis of research on staff development. *Educational Leadership, 38*(2), 182–185.

Military.com.education.training. Retrieved from http://usmilitary.about.com/od/educationtraining/United_States_Military_Education_and_Training_Programs.htm.

Murray, C. (1989). In search of the working poor. In R. C. Rist (Ed.), *Policy issues for the 1990s,* vol. 9 (pp. 975–1003). New Brunswick, NJ, and London: Transaction Press.

Rousseau, J. J. (1772). *Consideration on the government of Poland.* Edison, NJ: Transaction Press.

Silverberg, M., Warner, E., Fong, M., & Goodwin, D. (2004). *National assessment of vocational education: Final report to the US Congress.* Washington, DC: US Department of Education. Retrieved from /www2.ed.gov/rschstat/eval/sectech/activities.html.

Sparks, D. (1994). A paradigm shift in staff development. *Journal of Staff Development, 15*(4), 26–29.

Sparks, G. M. (1983, November). Synthesis of research on staff development for effective teaching. *Educational Leadership,* 65–72.

Tight, M. (2000). *Key concepts in adult education and training,* 2nd ed. London & New York: Routledge-Taylor & Francis.

US Department of Education, National Center for Education Statistics (2007). *The Condition of Education 2007* (NCES 2007–064),

Zinn, L. (1990). Identifying your philosophical orientation. *Adult learning methods: A guide to effective instruction.* Malabar, Florida: Krieger Publishing Company.

8

Health Education Centers: Teaching for Wellness

Introduction

On September 14, 2011, a 20-month-old toddler, Samyah Bailey, was caught in the middle of a gang gun battle on Staten Island, NY. A gunshot went through her skull, causing the doctors to remove her left eye. Emergency surgery and treatment were performed, saving her life but leaving her disfigured. Lack of health insurance for Samyah and her family made it necessary for family and friends to host fund-raisers to pay for her medical bill and living expenses.

Saymah's father said, "It's hard right now, even after that, trying to find housing, it's just hard living, life is hard in general. But my baby is alive and strong, and we've got help and support" (www.newyorknews.com).

In this example, clearly Saymahs's family is uninsured and must rely on the community to raise money to make her whole. Community involvement, financial support, and education are the processes that often step in to assist their residents when other means are inaccessible.

The United States faces a health-care crisis for both elderly and youth, especially those who live near or below the poverty level. The response to this crisis has been attempts to develop a universal care program, thus providing health assurance for all. President Obama breaks his health-care reform plan into three parts, saying that it would build "upon the strengths of the U.S. health care system."

The three parts are as follows:

1. Quality, Affordable, and Portable Health Coverage For All.
2. Modernizing the US Health-care System to Lower Costs and Improve Quality.
3. Promoting Prevention and Strengthening Public Health Services.

The US economy has continued to decline over the last several years, and unemployment has increased. If the drop is sustained, the number of uninsured will increase, raising the barrier to quality health care for millions of Americans. The costs of health care in this country are increasing. According to Strunk and Cunningham (2002), "Rising health care costs may prompt some employers to drop health benefits or pass on more costs to workers,...leading to a severe nursing shortage, an undersupply of doctors in certain areas, and then providers dropping out of health plan networks" (www.hschange.org).

Census data from the Center on Budget and Policy Priorities (2005) show the number of uninsured Americans to be at an all-time high. The 46 million Americans who are uninsured, including 8.3 million children, will likely get worse care, as economy worsens and unemployment increases.

While the need for universal health care is vital to the health of the country, the vitriolic responses to President health-care Obama's proposal put into question where the interest lies for those in power? The political divide is so deep that implementation and delivery of universal, fair health provision to all—or more people—seems improbable in the near future. And physician's political views on the plan vary, but consensus from the American Medical Association (AMA) is that the Patient Protection and Affordability Care Act (PPACA) does reform the US health-care system effectively. In a survey by Jackson Healthcare of doctors' opinion of the new proposed laws, physician respondents, "the majority considered themselves knowledgeable or *very* knowledgeable about the act and gave PPACA an average grade of D" (Jackson Healthcare, 2010).

The result has been a withdrawal of long-term health care for people with chronic illnesses and disabilities. Kathleen Sebelius, the Secretary of Health and Human Services, concluded, "the premiums would be too high and that healthy people would not sign up...and we have not found a way to make class work at this time" (Pear, 2011).

In addition, Kathy J. Greenlee, the assistant secretary of US Department of Health and Human Services, in charge of the program, said: "We do not have a viable path forward. We will not be working further to implement the Class Act" (Pear, 2011, p. 11). So, where can the poor go to receive preventative and curative treatment, and in turn be prepared for success in education and employment?

This chapter will examine the need for primary and preventative health care for children and adults who live at or near the poverty line. It will examine the drain on society economically and socially because of poor health care. The development of health-care centers—that treat and educate the poor and others in need—can (1) fill the health insurance gap, (2) teach families about healthier lifestyles, and (3) improve children's attendance and success in school—and thus increase the promise of more opportunities for better employment.

Connecting Health, Education, and Employment

The connection between health, education, and employment fulfillment is a foregone conclusion. According to a study by Ross and Wu (1995), three categories are affected by a healthy or unhealthy body and mind: These work and economic conditions include:

1. Work and economic conditions
2. Social-psychological resources, and
3. Healthier lifestyle. (pp. 719–720)

Examining the three effects may help us to find how well-educated people have better chances for full-time employment, with higher salaries and better retirement and health benefits. These conditions often translate into economic comfort and less hardship. Well-educated people have social-psychological resources, including great social support, sense of personal control, and economic resources. Last, well-educated people live healthier lifestyles. They are better informed of potential sickness, have greater access to primary care, and are more likely to exercise, eat a healthy diet, and refrain from smoking or drinking to excess.

Children—the future for advancement and social mobility—are also the most fragile when it come to health-related issues. Case and Paxson (2006), analyzing three British data sets, found "growing evidence that health in childhood is a determinant of educational attainment, which, in turn, affects adults' employment opportunities and wages" (p. 3).

Also, children's health has influences on their economic success, for, first, poor health diminishes success in educational attainment, which then, second, affects opportunities for better employment, and it often determines health conditions in adulthood, which can have impact on an individual's ability to find a good-paying job. As Case and Paxson (2006) point out, "Children with poor health may be less school-ready than other children...may miss more days and may complete fewer years in schooling over-all. Poorer schooling could limit their earning potential, quality of life, and possible health levels as adults" (p. 10).

Social scientists see education as the most influential investment a country can make in its citizens, improving skills, wages, economic well-being, birth control, hygiene, living conditions, health of children and adults, and life expectancy (Summers, 1992). However, with weak political support for a US national health program—a lack of commitment on the part of physicians, and no real voice for the poor and underserved—how can we overcome the problem of a growing incidence of poor health leading to nonproductiveness, suffering, and social stagnation?

Furthermore, according to the National Health Center, the United States is facing a shortage of qualified physicians and dentists to serve an increasing demand of a growing older and underinsured population. Attention to children's health can begin to ameliorate the issues of educational failure, adult unemployment, and economic dependency. Passing and implementing policies to prevent and treat illnesses early on can improve economic status in adulthood, contribute to the GDP, and improve social mobility to higher and healthier standards of living and quality of life.

Area Health Education Centers

Area health education centers go relatively unnoticed, but serve those unable to gain access to primary care physicians and treatment clinics supported by health insurance. The program actually began in 1971 and intended to serve *rural areas* where few doctors practiced. Medical students, residents, and nurse trainees became the main staffing sources supported by public funding and state hospitals. The initiative began as a result of needs in these more-isolated areas, and the hope was to incentivize medical trainees and interns to start their own practice in high-needs areas.

The main goal, according to Tara Kaprowy (2011), is "to link students in all types of health professions to rural and underserved training sites such as clinic, hospitals and physicians offices" (*Kentucky Health News Online*). The role of Area Health Education Center is to serve communities where residents have little or no insurance and have limited access to quality health care. Stimulating interest in the health professions begins in high schools, initiating students through volunteer work and training in clinics and promoting further education in all areas of need.

The effort to reach communities in high-needs urban and rural areas helped establish funding initiated from the PPACA of 2010. The Act, signed into law on July 6, was intended to expand health insurance to all Americans, including the 45 million uninsured in the United States. Even so, in a recent court ruling, the Act was declared unconstitutional, leaving the status quo of the uninsured intact. The rulings in four different federal courts have tied, two *for* the act and two *against* it. Thus, the law is still in limbo and meanwhile, 45 million Americans remain without health insurance.

While the debate over the PPACA continues to rage in the House and Senate, physicians voices have also commented on their obligations to address "societal health policy issues." Dr. Collen Ryan et al. (2009) reported, based on a survey, that while primary care physicians generally supported limits on reimbursement in the plan, specialty doctors "were all significantly less likely to favor reform that reduces reimbursement" (p. 58). While the status of Obama's health-care proposal rages on, area health clinics have tried to serve those most in need.

Serving the Medically Neglected

Community health centers are located in areas where low-income, medically underserved, and uninsured residents live. According to Gulfcoast North Area Health Education Center, Inc., "Over 1,000 community, migrant, and homeless health centers serve 3,600 urban and rural communities in every state and territory" (n.p.). Answering the need of poor families as the decade-old debate drags on, community health centers try to answer the need with primary care. Educating the poor concerning their right to health insurance or how to negotiate the Medicaid system is part of the community center's goal.

The nation's first community health centers began in 1965, as part of President Lyndon B. Johnson's "war on poverty" and economic growth plan. The continued increase in the number of health centers has flourished, but their existence is not highly visible. Even so, by the year 2008, 17 million of the underserved and medically neglected have been provided health care throughout the United States.

Today, community health centers have become an integral part of primary care systems in both urban and rural communities that provide a quality medical care. Many health-care facilities operate during hours that force low-wage earners to choose either a health-care visit and lose of their daily wages, or to neglect the immediacy of their medical problems. In some rural areas, moreover, the distance to a health-care facility causes hardship in travel time and available access. The community health center attempts to locate itself in the most vulnerable areas, structuring services based on a community's needs. Planning for flexible hours, translation for non-English speaking clients, and keeping open on weekends allow for easier access and better availability.

Technology, too, has transformed the opportunity to be seen by specialists in distant locations. For those who volunteer their services, online video-conferencing can assist local community health-care workers to diagnose and treat more difficult cases long-distance.

The Community Center as Educator

New York City boasts a school-based health and family planning center that is of interest. Located in Washington Heights in upper Manhattan—serving residents from there and high-needs areas such as Inwood and Harlem—the center is associated with the Mailman School of Public Health Department of Population and Family Health at Columbia University.

The center collaborates with local public schools, the department of pediatrics, obstetrics, and other specialty areas including dentistry and ophthalmology. The Center for Community Health and Education (CCHE) states as its mission:

> To improve the health of adolescents, women and men by providing high-quality and comprehensive medical, mental health education services. CCHE advances service innovations through community partnerships, teaching and advocacy. Patients are treated with dignity, courtesy, and confidentiality regardless of ability to pay.

The center's outreach to educate parents and adolescents include preventative measures for HIV and STDs and unwanted pregnancies through after-school science clubs and lessons. Taught by undergraduate medical and graduate students from Columbia University, the object is to increase awareness and self-advocacy in prevention. Programs in elementary and middle school emphasize healthy diets and exercise through active participation in after-school activities. Obesity and morbidity are most prevalent in low-income communities. Promoting, demonstrating, and creating an environment, where a culture of healthy lifestyles are emphasized, are the purposes of the program for children and community.

Perhaps, the most important programs are area health clinics, needed to implement a medical literacy effort for their clients. Understanding illnesses, medications, dosage, side effects, and symptoms of illnesses could prevent life-threatening errors due to ignorance and bad treatment. Teaching self-advocacy for health is an all-important criterion for a healthier society, be it prevention or knowledge of responsible treatment when an illness does occur. Educating the poor, adolescents, and those who might engage in high-risk behaviors can reduce the cost of health care and result in upward social mobility.

Health centers for primary care and education are set up in every state, serving communities' needs. These initiatives work to develop more *teaching health centers,* allowing opportunities for residents to (1) have training, (2) develop skills, (3) gain experience in the health professions, and (4) further the education not be available to them otherwise. The initiative, while worthy of support and further development, does not help the ever-increasing number of Americans without basic health care or access except through emergency room care.

Community Centers: Children and the Unwed Mother

Adrienne Nicole LeBlanc (2003), a literary journalist, followed two romances in the Bronx, NY, through gang affiliations, drugs, prison, and poverty. As of the ten years, with LeBlanc living with the families, unfolded, she wrote about the struggles of two single women, searching for meaning through love, drugs, babies, and prison. The main character in the story is a graphic example of the outcome for too many young girls who are brought up in an environment with a lack of education, and weak family and community support. The results in LeBlanc's true stories were four babies born to young women with four different absentee fathers.

According to the National Vital Statistics (1998), nearly 60 percent of all teens who become pregnant are living in poverty at the time of giving birth. Estimated are that during the first 13 years of parenthood, adolescent mothers earn an average of only $5,600 annually, less than half of the amount to be at poverty level. Thus, teenage mothers have a 50 percent chance of becoming dependent on welfare. The children brought up in these environments are often medically uninsured, have little preventative care, and miss many school days from sickness.

Thus, they too often fall behind in school—as the pattern of absenteeism and poor school performance are repeated, as they grow older. More uninsured children live in single-parent households with young unwed mothers. The poverty rate for children and their young mother is far greater than any other group in the United States.

For the sixth consecutive year, the number of Americans without health insurance has risen, according to new US Census Bureau data. With 60.2 percent fewer Americans having employer-based coverage since 2006, the figures for uninsured children—the most fragile cohort—had risen from 10.9 percent to 11.7 percent in one year (2006–2007). According to Executive Director Dr. George Benjamin, FACP, of the American Public Health Association (2006–2007), "children who are uninsured are more than three times less likely to have seen a doctor in the last year, and have a higher incidence of preventable diseases than insured children."

In another study conducted by the National Poverty Center at the University of Michigan, the impact of poverty on different subgroups revealed, "Poverty rates are highest for families headed by single women, particularly if they are black or Hispanic. In 2010, 31.6 percent of households headed by single women were poor, while 15.8 percent of households headed by single men and 6.2 percent of married couple households lived in poverty."

Outcomes for teen and unwed mothers often include poor health, lack of good education, and heavy reliance on welfare or low-wage earnings. For the children born to these mothers, they often have poor health, lower educational achievement, and prospect for future employment is bleak.

Without intervention and education, perpetuation of the same conditions has been documented. "The evidence shows that children born to teenage mothers are more likely to experience a range of negative outcomes in later life and are more likely, in time, to become teenage parents themselves—perpetuating the disadvantage that young parenthood brings from one generation to the next" (Ermisch and Pevalin 2003, p. 3).

Instituting new policies and better practices can successfully change these outcomes. Policy makers need to understand the cost to society, both economically and socially, that result from teen pregnancies and births. The cost to taxpayers is approximately $7 billion annually in lost revenues and expenses associated with health care, foster care, criminal justice, and public assistance related to teenagers' pregnancy and childbearing.

Policies and practices to prevent teens from premature motherhood should begin with better education of children in schools and community centers in areas with increased numbers of teen pregnancies. Support services must be provided, once the pregnancy is known, to assure good prenatal health, education on childcare, assistance for housing, and continued schooling and training for future employment.

The relationship between academic failure and teen pregnancy is strong; teens who are doing well in school, are positively motivated, and see future promise for employment and social stability are less likely to become pregnant in their teens. Relationships with teachers, school personnel, and peers can have a positive influence on the behavior of these adolescents.

Reintroducing more nonacademic programs, such as vocational and skill-based programs, can help alleviate the high failure, dropout, and pregnancy rate among teens. Reforming our education system to adopt a more-inclusive model for all types of learners will decrease some of the high-risk behaviors associated with school failure. Including sex education classes and creating school-based health clinics will help avoid unwanted pregnancies—and provide support and parenting education when pregnancy does occur.

The elimination of the school nurse, due to budget cuts, has been a great loss for the public school system. School nurses provide educational support, counseling, and community resources for the teen mother. Understanding without being negative or judgmental, the school nurse can help the teen *mother* receive the training and support; and the *infant* to get the prenatal health, afterbirth care, and encouragement for continuing education and positive parenting.

In a study done by Strunk (2008), a meta-analysis on the effectiveness of school-based clinics on outcomes of teenage pregnancies from 1997 to 2006 was measured, including the young mother's:

- absenteeism,
- dropout rates,
- low grade-point averages,
- repeat pregnancy rates,
- needed parenting skills,
- immunization rates in infants,
- social problem-solving skills,
- responsiveness to infants.

Results of this program indicate improved effectiveness and positive outcomes on pregnancies, and better parenting as well as educational outcomes for the mothers. Perhaps most important, the evidence from Strunk's meta-analysis showed that "the most important components of a school-based program were counseling, healthcare, health teaching, and child development education" (p. 15).

Community support programs vary according to location (the state) and resources. For example: "Second Chance" housing, supported by the U. S. Department of Housing and Urban Development, is a community-based program assisting teen mothers by affording them a safe place to live, and collaboration with others in their situation. The program provides information about childcare, further education and a track to eventual independence (http://www. livestrong.com/article/124754-programs-teen-moms/#ixzz1bW1RkQfI).

An Oregon based program, "Insight Teen Parent Program" offers services to teen parents, mothers and fathers, in finding affordable housing, continuing their education and employment possibilities. Medical care and support for the new babies is given and the families are followed to offer continued support and education. (http://www.livestrong.com/article/124754-programs-teen-moms/#ixzz1bW1qHhU4).

Lipman and Boyle (2003) conducted a research project to determine the efficacy of a social support and education program for single mothers. Instituting a randomized trial of a community-based program, the researchers recruited 116 mothers of children, 3–6 years of age for the study. Random assignments were made to participate in a 10-week program consisting of group sessions of one and a half hours weekly. The groups focused on social support and education running parallel to their children's activity group. The mothers were also given a list of community resources and the option to continue in-group sessions at the end of the trial period.

Assessment of the efficacy of the groups was measured from baseline data at the beginning of the study, immediately following the sessions, and then three and six months later. Self-reported outcome measures included mother's mood, self-esteem, social support, and parenting. Improvements in all categories were noted but long-term follow-up showed attenuation in each.

While the long-term results weakened with time, community-based support for single mothers proved that ongoing support and education would be beneficial to the mothers, and in turn, would then benefit their children. Children living with mothers who have higher confidence, better self-esteem, and improved parenting skills have a better chance of success in schools, and greater potential upward social mobility.

The most well-known intervention for young teen mothers and their children has been the research done in *Abecedarian Project*. Begun in 1972, the study has followed early childcare and education through 2007. McLaughlin et al., reported (2007) on the efficacy and success of the program beginning at infancy and followed through adulthood. Children and teen mothers were selected on the basis of High Risk Index scores and then randomized for inclusion in intervention or control groups.

One hundred and eleven infants and their mothers were selected, 57 in the experimental and 54 in the control groups. The following are indicators of the program's intensity during the eight years of intervention, five in preschool and three in primary school:

- The intervention groups receiving preschool treatment had higher IQ-skill development scores than those in the control group.
- At age, 50 percent of children with no intervention were retained, compared with 38 percent of those receiving interventions.
- Ages 8, 12, 15, and 21 of those with preschool intervention received higher overall Weschler Intelligence (IQ) test scores.
- Age 21 found 36 percent attending four-year college compared to 14 percent of those in the control group.

The education of the infants and young children was reinforced with parental education for their teen mothers. They were given specific support and instructions year round, helping the young mothers succeed in parenting and also in finding more meaningful employment to support their families. The outcomes of early intervention programs have demonstrated a range of benefits for the children and their families in high-risk communities: educationally, behaviorally, economically, and health related.

To convince policy and decision makers, we first need to convince leaders, not only about their moral obligation to the families that struggle to break the hold of poverty, but also about the forthcoming economic benefits to society and the country at large. The evidence of the benefits of early childhood programs—along with teen mother education—has been documented in several research studies from the 1960s to the present. Ready access to three well-known studies: the Chicago CPC Program, the High Scope Perry Preschool Program, and the Carolina Abecedarian Project, all present evidence of positive outcomes for the majority of children and their mothers.

Temple and Reynolds (2007), for example, speak of the results of the three preschool programs as follows: "The magnitude of estimated effects varied across the three studies...the impact was large with significantly lower rates of special education services (40–60%), participation was linked to higher rates of school completion up to age 27...higher rates of postsecondary and college attendance." (p. 132).

The largest return for teen mother participants was linked to the Abecedarian Project in employment and earnings. Table 8.1 shows the cost and benefits (in dollars) per participant in 2002 for the three

Table 8.1 Cost Analysis per Program

Cost and Benefits	High Scope Perry Preschool	Child-Parent Centers	Abecedarian Project
Program Cost $			
Average program Participant:	$15,844	$7,384	$35, 864
One year of Participation:	9759	4,856	13,900
Program Benefits $			
Total Benefits:	138,486	74,981	135,546
Net Benefits (benefits-costs):	122,642	67,595	99, 682
Total Benefits per Dollar invested:	8.74	10.15	3.78
Public benefit per Dollar invested:	7.16	6.87	2.69

Source: Retrieved from Temple and Reynolds (2007).

Note: Costs are program expenditures and for comparability were converted to 2002 dollars using the Consumer Price Index.

Table 8.2 Preschool Program Effects Related to Economic Benefits

Outcome Variable		Program Group Measure N		No Program Group Measure N	
Education Effects (children)					
IQ Stanford Binet	age 3	101	50	84	48
IQ(McCarthey)	age 4.5	101	49	91	46
IQ (WISC-R)	age 15	95	48	90	44
Reading (WJ)	age 15	94	48	88	44
Math Ach. (WJ)	age 15	93	48	82	44
Retention Rate	age 15	31%	48	55%	44
Special Services by	grade 9	25%	48	48%	44
HS Graduation by	age 19	67%	54	51%	51
College Enrolled by	age 21	36%	53	13%	51
Employment Effects at participant's age of 54 months (teenage parents)					
Teenage mothers and Postsecondary training		46%	13	13%	15
Teen mothers and self Supporting		70%	13	58%	15
Teenage mothers and Additional births		23%	13	40%	13

Note: Differences are significant at the .05 level of confidence. Definitions: WISC-R is the Wechsler Intelligence Scale for Children Revised; WJ is the Woodcock Johnson Psycho-Educational Battery, Part 2: Test of Academic Achievement, McCarthy CGI is the McCarthy General Cognitive Index. Community health and education projects have lasting effects. Employment rates are higher; and according to a study by the Frank Porter Graham Child Development Institute, maternal earning, based on actual data at ages 32, 35, and 41, are reported at $43,030, (in 2002 dollars). Policy makers should do the math; and thus add in the dollar value and human capital contribution to the standards rhetorically set for all citizens. Adding tax dollars—and deleting losses in term of health, joblessness, and incarceration—could certainly be the impetus to refocus our obligation to the poor and society.

preschool programs: ages of participants for the study were 27, 21, and 22 years old, respectively (Chicago CPC, High Scope Perry Preschool, Abecedarian Project).

According to the report by Temple and Reynolds (2007), the costs, while different for each program, all exceeded the initial investment. The present value of the total economic benefits per participant, both measured and projected over the life course, ranged from $74,981 to $138, 486.

Table 8.2 is an indictor of the connection of health, educational attainment, and the welfare and earning potential for children and adults participating in an intense, all-inclusive early childhood program.

Conclusion

This chapter has covered the importance—morally, ethically, and economically—of assisting and breaking the cycle of poverty prevalent in the

United States. The introduction of more health education centers, that are more easily accessible, will improve the lives of children and adults. Understanding the cognitive benefits for the young of healthy bodies and environments will lead to better school performance and educational gain. Perpetuation of the same dependency on the welfare system cannot be changed until the community changes.

Empowering children to learn, mothers to parent, and employment opportunities for adults should be the main goals. Community health education centers are in need of support, getting more resources and tools to provide the assistance to their community members. Currently, single-parent families in poor neighborhoods suffer from lack of education, greater depression, cognitive loss due to environmental factors, drug and alcohol abuse, more crimes, and higher rates of imprisonment.

Community centers invite all neighborhood residents to seek help and to learn the basic tenets of healthy living, and to provide training for possible employment. The benefits of health for children's attendance and learning are well-documented, as sick, hungry, and neglected children cannot be expected to focus on the necessary instruction for academic gains.

Several programs such as High Score Perry Preschool, The Chicago Early Childhood Program, and Abecedarian Project have all documented success rates for helping young mothers, and their children become healthier, more well-educated, and self-sustaining over decades of study and follow-up. Community centers that focus on child and parent have a better chance of breaking the cycle of poverty, as evidenced by statistical data. (Campbell and Ramey, 2007).

The fight over cost for universal health care as a political issue is misdirected in focus, lacking the knowledge of the benefits of a healthy, educated, and well-working society. Adding to the tax base, from those currently on assistance, increases the possibility for better schools, a healthier, happier citizenry, and a productive, more economically successful country.

References

Benjamin, G., MD, Executive Director (2006–2007) *APHA (American Public Health Association)*.

Campbell, F. A., & Ramey, C. T. (2007). Critical issues in cost effectiveness in children's first decade. Paper presented at National invitational conference of the early childhood research collaborative. St. Paul: University of Minnesota.

Case, A., & Paxson, C., (2006, Fall). Children's health and mobility. *Opportunity in America, 16*(2).

CCHE (Center for Community Health and Education), New York City.

Center on Budget and Policy Priorities (2005). Number and Percentage of Americans who are Uninsured climbs Again in 2005. Retrieved from www.cbpp.org/cms

Ermisch, J., & Pevalin, D. (2003). Who has a child as a teenager? *Institute for Social and Economic Research,* University of Essex. Retrieved from www.iser.essex.uk/pubs/workpaps/pdf/2003–30.pdf

Jackson Healthcare (2010) *PPACA.* Retrieved from www.jacksonhealthcare.com.

Kaprowy, T. (2011). *Kentucky Health News.* Retrieved from kyhealthnews.blogspot.com.

LeBlanc, A. N. (2003). *Random family: Love, drugs, trouble, and coming of age in the Bronx.* New York: Scribner Publishing.

Lipman, E. L., & Boyle, M. H. (2003, May 23). *Barriers to services promoting child emotional, behavioral and social health.* Retrieved from http://www.child-encyclopedia.com/documents/lipman- boyleANGxp.pdf.

Livestrong Community Programs. Retrieved from http://www.livestrong.com.

McLaughlin, A. E., Campbell, F. C., Pungello, E. P., & Skinner, M. (2007). Depressive symptoms in young adults: The influences of the early home environment and early educational childcare. *Child Development, 78,* 746–756.

National Poverty Center (2010). University of Michigan.

National Vital Statistics (1998).

Paddock, B., Kerry, W. & Doyle, J. (2011). Samyah Bailey, Just Shy of Her Second Birthday, Loses Eye after Getting Struck by Stray Bullet. September 14. Retrieved from www.newyorknews.com

Pear, R. (2011, October 14). Health law to be revised by ending a program. *New York Times, pp. 10–11.*.

Ross, C. E., & Wu, L. (1995). The links between education and health. *American Sociological Review, 60*(5), 719–745.

Ryan, M., Antiel, M. A., Farr, A. Curlin, M. D. James, K., & Tilburt, J. C. M.D., M.P . (2009, October 1). Physician's beliefs and U. S. health care reform—A national survey. *New England Journal of Medicine, 361*(23), 57–62.

Strunk, B. C., & Cunningham, P. (2002). In Green L. & S. Sergei (Eds.), *Providing timely access to medical care: A queuing model.* New York: Columbia University, Graduate School of Business.

Strunk, J. A. (2008). The effect of school-based clinics on teenage pregnancy and parenting outcomes: An integrated literature review. *The Journal of School Nursing, 24*(1), 13–20.

Summers, L. (1992). The most influential investment. *Scientific American, 270*,132.

Temple, J. A., & Reynolds, A. J. (2007). Benefits and cost of investments in preschool education:. Evidence from child-parent centers and related programs. *Economics Education Review, 26*(1), 126–144.

9

Health, Education, and the Community

Introduction: A Historical Perspective

In times past, schools served as the center of the community along with religious institutions and local businesses. The natural geography of neighborhoods encouraged the use of many of the school facilities, including playing fields for local residents, and conference and central meeting places for community interests and concerns. The integration of the entire community and its inhabitants often made schools a central focal point, supported by local boards made up of residents where their children attended.

A result of the local community school was the tendency to form partnerships that included all services within the school community: for example, health, education, and general welfare for the community at large. It set the principle for an integrated interest in academics, services, and support for the all residents living within its borders.

Perhaps the most important positive influence of the neighborhood school was its ability to unite families, to create connections and support that nurtured development and provided incentives to succeed. Services, created by the community, supported those in need, fostered feelings of belonging and safety, and generated opportunities for growth, productivity, and self-esteem.

On the flip side, Carl Kaestle (1983) traces "the staunchly defended American tradition of neighborhood schools to the 18th century. In rural America, these schools for white children belonged to and reflected the culture of the surrounding community" (p. 31).

In more rural settings, schools were often poorly funded and housed a mixed level of students in one-room buildings, where local officials appointed untrained teachers at miserly salaries. These schools survived into the twentieth century until urbanization increased the need for better professional training for teachers and the consolidation of schools into larger facilities. The intent of consolidation was both economic and educationally opportunistic, but spelled the end of neighborhood schools for many.

Urbanization clustered similar ethnic socioeconomic groups into neighborhoods and their schools. According to Lowe (2004), "The greater population density of cities ensured the long-term survival of urban neighborhood schools, but their uneven quality reflected the unequal distribution of power between neighborhoods differentiated by class and race" (p. 22). Urbanization, immigration, and the industrial revolution brought more responsibility to the schools for both education and socializing newcomers to the United States. Children of immigrants often lived in poverty and struggled to gain the learning and social skills expected at the time.

The needs in the communities were either met or not according to the status of the population in the "naturally" segregated schools and neighborhoods. Thus, history is repeating itself, through the racial and ethnic separation of the classes by socioeconomic means and perpetuating similar outcomes according to health, wealth, and opportunity (Coleman, 2007).

Back to Basics Reform

Today, with the end of busing and other efforts to desegregate schools and to increase the balance of ethnic and social-class groups, we have returned to the separate but equal mind-set first challenged in *Plessy v. Ferguson* in 1896. Neighborhood schools have once again become the status quo for policy makers with unequal funding, resources, and teacher quality. As Lowe (2004) asserts, "the current nationwide effort to restore neighborhood schools has little basis for promising excellent schools, but it can deliver racially separate ones" (n.p.).

The case for desegregation is now a dead issue, satisfying the white policy makers who control both funding and structure of the education system in the United States (Orfield and Eaton, 1996). This loss can be viewed with frustration or as an opportunity to develop community schools to serve the students and residents of the neighborhood. W. E. B. Du Bois (1935) reversed his stance on desegregation decades earlier, altering his view of providing excellence in education regardless of race or status. Du Bios explained:

> The Negro needs neither separate nor mixed schools. What he needs is Education. What he must remember is that there is no magic either in

mixed schools or segregated schools. A mixed school with poor unsympathetic teachers, with hostile public opinion, and no teaching of the truth concerning black folk is bad. A segregated school with ignorant placeholders, inadequate equipment, and poor salaries is equally bad. Other things being equal the mixed school is the broader more natural basis for the education of all youth. It gives wider contacts; it inspires greater self-confidence; and suppresses the inferiority complex. But other things seldom are equal, and in that case, Sympathy, Knowledge, and the Truth outweigh all that the mixed school can offer. (p. 335)

Knowledge and Power

Paolo Freire understood the power of knowledge and education. Fiercely unpopular with government officials in his native Brazil, Freire wrote *Politics of the Oppressed* (1985) to promote educating the lower classes: teaching them to advocate for their needs, understand their rights, and to use the power of their "voice" for change. Freire's theory of learning states that "the ability of humans to plan and shape the world for their future needs is what separates man from animals. The oppressed majority must be taught to imagine a better way so that they can shape their future and thereby become more human" (p. 94).

Without education, it is impossible to know what resources are available for health care, educational training, and better status for self-sustenance. Mirowsky, Ross, and Reynolds (2000), referring to Seaman's (1983) discussion of powerlessness, argued that "the link between socio-economic status and health may be explained in part by differential levels of perceived control, or beliefs in the extent which people can affect their outcomes by making particular choices." This lack of understanding prevents the impoverished from knowing the options that are available for them in a community or neighborhood for decent housing, educational quality, and resources.

Economic status had become the new segregation, separating the haves from the have-nots. The perpetuation of poor versus affluent communities and neighborhoods depends on parental education, occupation, and income status (Greenshaw, 1976). Children who grow up in more-affluent neighborhoods, where parents are well-educated, have better access to steady and good paying jobs, benefitting from a community that is prosperous with the resources to influence educational policies. Health care is consistent, with needed immunizations scheduled and chronic diseases prevented, treated, and controlled.

On the opposite side of town, housing is often in need of repair, lacking consistency in fundamentals: heat in the winter, hot water, and healthier living conditions. Schools are too often overcrowded, lacking the same resources found on the wealthier side of town; and teachers, while dedicated, are often new, inexperienced, and temporary (Brooks-Gunn, Duncan, and Aber, 1997). Health care is often neglected; and chronic diseases are treated only on an emergency basis.

The relationships of socioeconomic status, health, and educational attainment have been researched and analyzed by sociologists, epidemiologist, and educators. Experts have rarely agreed on whether genetics or environment is the cause for failure in schooling in poor neighborhoods. Leventhal and Brooks-Gunn (2002), for example, found in their research that neighborhoods do matter in educational achievement and well-being. The associations found suggest:

> Children living in high-income neighborhoods had higher cognitive ability and school achievement than those living in middle-income neighborhoods and children and adolescents living in low-income neighborhoods, had more mental and physical health problems than those living in middle income neighborhoods. (pp. 45–46)

Nature versus Nurture: Characteristics of Environment, Socioeconomic Status, and Family

Shonkoff and Phillips (2000), in a National Academy of Sciences report on child development, concludes "that it is an accretion of toxic stress and environmental risks—and not simply one factor, such as asthma or poor prenatal care, that impedes learning and well-being—which can lead to adult incarceration and diminished life chances so evident in statistics related to men and boys of color in the United States" (Shonkoff and Phillips, 2000, p. 7).

Neurons to Neighborhoods

The characteristics of a neighborhood—such as housing, access to businesses, transit, schools, and recreational resources—influence the climate within and outside of the family. Neighborhoods with few resources, unsafe housing, and environments often have a climate of distrust and isolation. Studies have shown that stressors caused by unsafe and unsavory climates are manifested in depression and lowered-cognitive functioning. A study reviewed by Gilman and Medway (2007) found that children who live under the stressors of poverty score at least four point lower on IQ tests and fall behind academically more than a year than children in more-affluent neighborhoods.

And a Harvard University study lead by Sampson (2007) determined: "For children, living in disadvantaged neighborhood appears to contribute to a detrimental effect on trajectories of verbal ability" (n.p.). Language and verbal abilities, the most important factors in learning, need to be developed in the early years of childhood to assure academic success, and exposure to poor language usage, dialect, and fewer opportunities to communicate with others can contribute to lower or failing achievement rates.

Sampson (2007) explained, "Even beyond their economic situation, children in neighborhoods of concentrated disadvantage are exposed to a myriad of social factors that can deflect developmental trajectories" (n.p.). Research by neuroscientists and others in the medical and scientific communities has concluded that the developing brain is altered by social environmental conditions. Understanding the impact of the environment can help in our quest to change certain factors for more positive outcomes.

These discussions need to take place to inform and react to a problem that affects nearly one in four children living in impoverished households.

The Community School: Neighborhood and Community Resource

How do we mobilize and educate residents in high-need neighborhoods to advocate change for themselves and their children? President Lyndon B. Johnson characterized racial inequality as a "seamless web." In a commencement address at Howard University on June 4, 1965, he stated:

> The root causes of inequality, he said, are "complex and subtle." A child's chances to prosper and fulfill his potential, Johnson said, depend not merely upon his attributes and perseverance but upon the social conditions in the society. Johnson characterized sources of racial inequality, as "a seamless web...They cause each other. They result from each other. They reinforce each other." Men and women of all races are born with the same range of abilities. But ability is not just the product of birth. Ability is stretched or stunted by the family that you live with, and the neighborhood you live in—by the school you go to and the poverty or the richness of your surroundings. It is the product of a hundred unseen forces playing upon the little infant, the child, and finally the man.

Improving the quality of schools can help to change the community and to create resources for positive development and outcomes for children, adolescents, and adult residents. Developing a partnership with care, trust, and respect can be a catalyst for a change. The school can be a community center where all have access to health and education, job training and childcare—a full-service facility open to all who live within the neighborhood.

Knowledge from the research on the developing child and his or her environment should provide the impetus to create and fund full-service schools. The alternatives—for example, dropouts, higher welfare costs, and more hospitalizations and incarceration of youth—are far more costly, depleting human capital productiveness and perpetuating problems from generation to generation.

Policy makers, in control of funding, should analyze the cost savings for full-service community schools. According to Sickmund, Sladky, and Kang (2008), states spent approximately $45.7 billion in 2007 to incarcerate 64,558 youth in juvenile facilities. The average cost for society in dollars approximates $241 per day, reaching $88, 000 per year. The annual cost on average per pupil in our school systems is $10,000–$16,000 (Cara Matthews, *The Ithaca Journal*). And the *Bureau of Justice Assistance* (Austin, Johnson, and Gregoriou, 2000) reported an increase of juvenile incarceration of 366 percent over a ten-year period. Certainly, spending the dollars in high-risk communities is a savings, not only in money, but also in human capital, resulting in an increase in revenue from productivity. It is time to educate, not to incarcerate.

The Full-Service School: Historical Perspective

The concept of a "community full-service school" is not new. John Dewey was an initiator of the community school more than one hundred years ago, advocating the application that all can learn (Boylston, 1991). He believed that "the significant thing is to make the school...a center of full and adequate social service...to bring it into the current of social life" (Dewey, 2007, p. 80), making the school into a major social center.

Even before Dewey, Jane Addams (1860–1935) the second woman to earn a Nobel Prize, founded the US Settlement House Movement, bringing health and educational services to immigrant neighborhoods in Chicago in 1889 (Benson, Havkavy, Johenek, and Puckett, 2009, p. 24). Addams was convinced that social circumstances interconnected with health, education, and welfare. She established Chicago's Hull House, offering college extension classes, social clubs, ethnic activities, health and legal services, and kindergarten for young learners. "These houses were often centers for labor union meetings, public forums, social science research and meeting centers for people advo-cating for social change" (Benson et al., 2009, p. 23).

During the Great Depression, with such limited resources, schools were seen as central facilities for multiple uses: leisure and/or recre-ational activities, health, counseling, and adult education. Schools remained open after the traditional hours to serve the needs of com-munities during this era and allowed community groups to problem solve, commiserate, and plan for the future. Johenek (1995) reported on the Benjamin James High School in East Harlem, New York City. Established in 1934 by an Italian immigrant, the all-boys school became a community center to address the social issues of poor housing, sanita-tion, and diverse group relations. According to Johenek (2009), "This was the first model that made the school 'the coordinator' of social ser-vices" (p. 24).

The 1960s brought the Great Society under President Lyndon Johnson, developing the Elementary and Secondary Education Acts (ESEA) and providing education for the neediest students. Head Start was created to promote readiness for young children, by addressing the educational, health, nutritional, and social needs of children. The involvement of gov-ernment acknowledged that schools alone could not address the causes, effects, and problems of social poverty.

James S. Coleman's "Equality of Educational Opportunity" (2007) addressed the external elements that impact the development of the human condition; family, neighborhood, peer influence, and economic conditions. Coleman (1926–1995) asserts that these external influences have more to do with educational attainment than the time spent in the classroom. This principle, perhaps, was an impetus for the passage of more current legislation that caused states to legislate the creation of community schools.

Where We Are: The Need for Community Schools

The nation's economic crisis has exacerbated the inequity in health, education, and welfare. Job losses and home foreclosures have affected everyone, with a deepening effect on those in the lower-socioeconomic strata of society. Homelessness, dangers, and hunger have increased as the country struggles to manage the fiscal downturn. The national agen-das have been politically skewed along party lines and special interests.

According to the American Psychological Association (2010), the child poverty rate has risen from 18 percent in 2007 to 19 percent in 2009, with trends increasing. African American, Black, and Hispanic children were more than twice as likely to live in impoverished conditions (Walker, 1996). And 53 percent of children with immigrant parents, and 42 percent with single mothers are living in neighborhoods that are physically, mentally, and educationally neglected.

The impact on student achievement is profound, as the dropout rate is ten times higher than the national average, perpetuating the conditions of poverty, crime, and physical and mental health problems.

Going to court and to jail are too often the results of a poor home and community environment, a lack of educational attainment, and few or no prospects for employment. The incarceration rate for under-18 children continues to increase; and instead of effecting change through imprisonment, recidivism was at an astounding 67.5 percent rate at a cost of $68,747,203,00 annually in the nation in 2010. According to the Bureau of Justice Statistics, "The number the number of youth under 18 confined in adult prisons has more than doubled in the past decade...Approximately 107,000 youth (younger than 18) are incarcerated on any given day."

Table 9.1 presents the result of disconnected youth living in conditions that lead to imprisonment instead of educational attainment:

The increase of youth placed in adult prisons has grown from 8,090 in 1998 to 11,300 in 2009, according to the Bureau of Justice. The cost

Table 9.1   Juveniles in Adult Jails, 1983–1998

Year	Total Adults in Jail	All Male	All Female	Juvenile
1983	221,815	206,163	15,652	1,736
1984	233,018	216,275	16,743	1,482
1985	254,986	235,909	19,077	1,627
1986	272,736	251,235	21,501	1,708
1987	294,092	270,172	23,920	1,788
1988	341,843	311,594	30,299	1,676
1989	393,248	356,050	37,198	2,250
1990	403,019	365,821	37,198	2,301
1991	424,129	384,628	39,501	2,350
1992	441,780	401,106	40,674	2,804
1993	455,600	411,500	44,100	4,300
1994	479,800	431,300	48,500	6,700
1995	499,300	448,000	51,300	7,800
1996	510,400	454,700	55,700	8,100
1997	559,974	498,670	59,296	9,105
1998	584,372	520,581	63,791	8,090
% change between 1983 and 1998	+ 143%	+153%	+308%	+366%

Source: Bureau of Justice Statistics, 2010, p. 48.

to society—monetarily and loss of human capital—is high, with negative consequences politically, economically, and qualitatively.

Poor communities are losing too many of their youth. They need assistance in bringing together programs with social networks that intervene at the earliest stages, possibly breaking the cycle that persists in denigration and despair.

Communities need to come together, to create centers to help address all the issues encompassing poverty, and to begin to break the cycle of health, education, and welfare neglect. The school, a facility already present in the neighborhood, is the perfect place to build community, and to address the barriers for success and productivity. The Coleman Report (1966) asserted that external environments, including the home, neighborhood, and peer networks, have a greater impact on student academics achievement than schools alone. Apparently, all data and research indicate that school, as a separate entity from the neighborhood, cannot address all the social ills plaguing the poor.

Full Service, Community/Neighborhood Schools

Today, many traditional schools are unionized and standardized. Hours for learning are set; prescribed lessons are often mandated to pass tests that have little or no application to daily life. Chronological ages are prerequisites for entry and exit, and after-school activities rely on the funding from state and local school boards. Extra resources for enrichment (music and the arts) depend on the wealth of the district, leaving poorer communities often without it.

Statistically, we are falling behind academically on internationally ranked tests with an increasing dropout rate. And we often are spending more on incarcerated youth than those attending school. The national agenda on education is ill-conceived and failing. Money spent on social programs has become a hot political issue dividing the country into factions. The billions spent might be drastically reduced if an investment is made in community schools and full-service programs that serve the social, health, and educational needs of the poor.

Full-Service Schools

Today, too many children come to school with problems of hunger, neglect, illness, addiction, and abuse, instead of just their backpacks. How can the school become the networking system to begin ameliorating the causes of social and academic failure? Acknowledging that schools (teachers and staff alone) cannot meet the needs of students with multiple risks associated with poverty, institutional changes, and program reform must focus on the whole child; his/her family, neighborhood, and social structure (Dryfoos, 1995; Flaxman and Passow, 1995). Rigsby, Reynolds and Wang (1995) assert that "referred to as the 'integrated,' 'collaborative,' 'coordinated,' or 'school-linked' services movement, its goal is to harness the resources of family, school, and community to create contexts that support students' learning success by meeting the physical and social wellness needs of students and their families" (p. 11).

Wang, Haertel, and Walberg (1994) demonstrated the influences prevalent in children and their potential as learners. Based on the results of 91 meta-analyses done in 1993, data shown in Table 9.2 are indicators of the contexts affecting possible success in school.

Inner-city schools have always been challenged to serve immigrants and other diverse populations. Today, in an attempt to meet the needs of increasingly diverse students, special programs have been developed to address specific categories. Although well-intentioned, these programs are not improving on the basic social as well as academic needs to assimilate families into the general structure of society.

Institutional changes require an approach that invests in a full operational program that supports school organization, curriculum, teacher education, and full community services responsive to the health, education, and welfare of children families and other adults in the neighborhood.

Policymakers, educators, and local government officials need to weigh the costs and wasted potential lost for the unwell, undereducated, and the impoverished. Reforming should help to create environments where children and their families contribute to, rather than are a burden on, the GNP.

The full-service school is a step in that contribution; providing full-service school expands beyond the traditional hours of operation from 8:00 a.m. to 3:00 p.m. Community members and residents can assist in

Table 9.2   Contexts Affecting Student Success, 1983

Average Influence	
Source/Context	*Average Influence on Learning Score*
Classroom practices	53.3
Home and community	51.4
Curriculum design and delivery	47.2
School-wide practices and policies	45.1
State and district policies	34.5

identifying what the needs of the neighborhood and community are and suggest how they can be met. Health and social services, educational workshops, support groups, and childcare are the main ingredients necessary in full-service schools. Community agencies become an integral part of such a facility that remains open after hours, on the weekends, and throughout the summer.

The community schools' movement is a national initiative dedicated to creating committed, lasting partnerships among schools and their neighborhoods. In California this initiative is best known as "Healthy Start," which works to bring schools, families, neighborhoods, public and private agencies, and business together to meet student and family's needs. It has served as the Healthy Start Field Office since 1992, providing orientation training and technical assistance to over eight-hundred grantees.

According to Dryfoos (1995), "needs related to physical and mental health, dentistry, social services, after school activities, and educational enrichment are addressed on-site" (p. 38). Community schools develop partnerships with other community resources and integrate services with academic support. Children and families receive physical and mental health support; academic remediation and classes are provided for parents to complete their GED. Open all day, in the evenings, and on the weekends, activities and opportunities are available for enrichment and support for social development.

The Coalition for Community Schools Program (CCSP) is described by the Children's Aid Society as

> combining the rigorous academics of a quality school with a wide range of vital in-house services, supports, and opportunities for the purpose of promoting children's learning and development. The community-school unites the most important influences in children's lives—school, families, and communities—to create a web of support that nurtures their development toward productive adulthood.

Utilizing the neighborhood school as the cog in the wheel, the process creates relationships among educators at the school, health and social service agencies, volunteer groups, families, businesses, and youth development organizations. Deborah Meier, *In Schools We Trust* (2002), demonstrated the possibilities of family- and youth-oriented schools. Benefitting from smaller environments that welcomed parents and promoted youth-adult partnerships, students from New York's East Harlem's Central Park East and the Mission School in Boston, had academic success based on involvement, trust, and caring. According to Deborah Meier, schools should be smaller, self-governing, as places of choice, so kids and their families feel that they are truly part of communities of learners.

The process for initiating and operating full-service schools depends upon the state grants and applications. Awards for the community coalition of schools range from $2,300,000 to $2,500,000 over a five-year period. The partners engaged in the grants vary from state to state. Consistent in each of the programs are the following: Identified low-wealth areas, poor academic results, other stress factors for families, and partners willing to participate in administering services.

Relying on competitive grants to receive funding is one fault in its policy. While those who start the initiative and talent to propose, write, and submit a grant have the intention of assisting poor families, too many students who might qualify are left behind without the possibility of receiving the services that they need to generate the chance for success. Acknowledging and using research from educational and scientific agencies, we must begin to implement institutional reform to address and treat the symptoms that deplete human capital and reduce reliance on costly subsidy programs.

Summary

We propose and support institutional change to transform our inner-city and high-needs schools into community centers that coalesce the social services and educational supports for whole neighborhoods. The schools will serve as the centers that invite participation and serve community needs. Schools would remain open after hours for a full evening of resource; would support academics through tutoring, homework assistance, technology availability, and childcare; and would sponsor recreational activities. Health services that include preventative and treatment options, along with dental and counseling services, would be available to meet the community's needs. Encouraging parents to finish school, train for employment, and improve their English fluency will together help families to become involved in a supportive interaction with each other to stabilize the family unit and the community as a whole.

Community/full service schools are not a new concept. They build partnerships and connect the school to community resources. Schools become the place where focusing on academics is just one purpose; health resources, training and adult education programs are likewise available and encouraged for all who reside in the community. Perhaps best described by the Coalition for Community Schools, these programs combine "the rigorous academics of quality school with a wide range of vital in-house services, supports, and opportunities for the purpose of promoting children's learning and development."

We must recognize that the multitude of adversities faced by families and children cannot be addressed by the school in its present form. The resources for health, education, family support, and well-being should connect if we are to begin to solve the problems—physical and mental— that impede learning and progress. Successful strategies have been implemented and documented through the US Department of Education and the American Educational Research Association. The research community now has a knowledge-base that can serve as models for successful partnerships between schools and communities.

Politicians need to put aside their bias, examine the research, do a cost analysis, and get on board for a proven system. The combination of national, state, and local agencies can change the outcomes for many children and families and in the long run, benefit the country economically and productively.

Let's study the successes, change the accountability measures, and share the responsibility for success for all children. If the goal is to eliminate the achievement gap—between rich and poor, we must provide the benefits of full-service institutions.

References

American Psychological Association (2010). *The effects of poverty, hunger, and homelessness on children and youth.* New York: The author.

Austin, J., Johnson, K. D., & Gregoriou, M. (2000). *Juveniles in adult prisons and jails: A national assessment.* Washington, DC: George Washington University.

Benson, L., Harkavy, I., Johenek, M., & Puckett, J. (2009). The enduring appeal of community schools. *The American Educator, 33*(2), 22–29, 47.

Boylston, J. A. (1991). *The middle works of John Dewey 1899–1924*, vol. 2 (pp. 80–93). Carbondale: Southern Illinois University Press.

Brooks-Gunn, J., Duncan, G. J., & Aber, J. L. (Eds.) (1997). *Neighborhood poverty* (2 vols.). New York: Russell Sage Foundation Press.

Bureau of Justice Statistics (2010). *Prisoners in 2009.* Washington, DC: US Department of Justice. December 2010 NCJ 231675.

Coleman, J. S. (2007). *Equality of educational opportunity study* (EEOS). Ann Arbor, MI: Inter-university Consortium for Political and Social Research.

———. (1966). *The Coleman Report. Equality of education opportunity.* Washington, DC: US Department of Health, Education and Welfare.

Dewey, J. (2007), *Experience in education.* New York: Simon & Schuster.

Dryfoos, J. G. (1995). *Full-service schools: A revolution in health and social services for children, youth, and families.* San Francisco, CA: Jossey-Bass.

Du Bois, W. E. B. (1935, July). Does the Negro need separate schools? *Journal of Negro Education 4*, 227–335.

Flaxman, E., & Passow, A. H. (Eds.) (1995). *Changing populations/changing schools: The*
94th yearbook of the national society for the study of education. Chicago: University of Chicago Press.

Freire, P. (1985). *The politics of the oppressed—Culture, power, and liberation.* Translated by Donaldo Macedo, New York: Bergin & Garvey.

Gilman, R., & Medway, F. J. (2007). Teachers' perceptions of school psychology: Comparisons of regular and special education teachers across four states. *School Psychology Quarterly, 22*, 145–161.

Greenshaw, W. (1976). *Watch out for George Wallace.* Englewood Cliff, NJ: Prentice-Hall.

Johenek, M. (2009). The enduring appeal of community schools. *The American Educator, 33*(2), 22–47.

———. (1995). *The public purposes of public education: The evolution of community-centered schooling at Benjamin Franklin High School, 1934-44.* Philadelphia: University of Pennsylvania.

Kaestle, C. F. (1983). Pillars of the republic: Common schools and American society,1780–1860. New York: Hill and Wang, 1983.

Leventhal, T., & Brooks-Gunn, J. (2002). A randomized study of neighborhood effects on low-income children's educational outcomes. Manuscript submitted for publication.

Lowe, R. (2004) *Originally, Rethinking Schools*, vol. 18, no. 3. Retrieved from http://www.rethinkingschools.org/archive/18_03/stra183.shtml.

Matthews, C. (2010). New York public schools top nation in per-pupil spending. *Ithaca Journal.* Retrieved from www.usatoday.com/news/… /2010–06–29-school-spending_htm.

Meier, D. (2002). *In schools we trust: Creating communities of learning in an era of testing and standardization.* Boston, MA: Beacon Press.

Mirowsky, J., Ross, C. E., & Reynolds, J. (2000). Links between social status and health status. *The Handbook of medical sociology.* New Jersey: Prentice Hall.

Orfield, G., & Eaton, S. E. (1996). Dismantling Desegregation: The Quiet Reversal of *Brown v.Board of Education.* New York: The New Press.

Rigsby, L. C., Reynolds, M. C., & Wang, M. C. (Eds.) (1995). *School-community connections: Exploring issues for research and practice.* San Francisco, CA: Jossey Bass.

Sampson, R. J. (2007). *Legitimacy and criminal justice: A comparative perspective.* New York: Russell Sage. Foundation.

Shonkoff, J. P., & Phillips, D. A. (2000). From neurons to neighborhoods: The science of early childhood. Washington, DC: The National Academies Press.

Sickmund, M., Sladky, T. J., & Kang, W. (2008). Census of juveniles in residential placement databook. Retrieved from http://ojjdp.ncjrs.gov/ojstatbb/cjrp/asp/State_Adj.asp; American Correctional Association, *2008 directory: Adult and juvenile correctional departments, institutions, agencies, and probation and parole authorities* (Alexandria, VA: American Correctional Association, 2008).

US Department of Health and Human Services (2010). National Center for Health Statistics. Washington, DC.

Walker, V. S. (1996). Their highest potential: An African-American school community in the segregated South. Chapel Hill : University of North Carolina Press

Wang, M. C., Haertel, G. D., & Walberg, H. J. (1994). Educational resilience in inner cities. In M. C. Wang, M. C. & E. W. Gordon (Eds.). *Educational resilience in inner-city America: Challenges and prospects* (pp. 45–72). Hillsdale, NJ: Lawrence Erlbaum.

Part III

Reconnecting Health, Education, and Welfare for the Common Good

This third section shows the strengths and advantages of reconnecting and improving the three fields and services, for the benefit of all. Using examples from the field, this section summarizes the examples and cases of how the wealth and income of families relates and influences their children's health and support from birth, if not before, and sets the conditions for growth, entry into schools, and their chances of good higher education and employment.

The issues in this book have major implications for twenty-first century families—their schools, health and welfare for the future. Better health and education, not only makes families more productive and prosperous, but also reduces the burden on society in educating and supporting them.

10

Connecting Early Childcare, Health, and School Preparation

Young children need good healthcare, socio-emotional support, and early exposure to ideas and concepts if they are to be prepared for school. Already, the American system has gone from being a 1-to-12 grade program, to kindergarten, and even prekindergarten to see that they are well cared for socially, intellectually, and physically from the start. This chapter interconnects early health-care programs, education and social experiences to growth, preparation for formal school, and long-term success.

Again, we see that families with resources provide all three: pediatric medical attention before and after birth, good social experiences early, such as play groups, social opportunities, and early preschool education. Good early childcare programs and early education benefit, not only the individual, but also the community and society as a whole. More productivity means better income and more consumption, which further fuels the economy and provides higher income tax that supports schools and other public services.

We show that wealth and income are related to education, in complex ways. More income can give parents more education options for their children; and a good education can open job and career options that in turn can often mean higher income. Well-being and quality of life cannot be attained without the basic environmental factors of health, physical, and mental, education for employment and sustenance, and community that fosters safety and support. Children—brought up in a positive climate with supportive families and resources to cover all the necessities outlined by Maslow's Hierarchy of needs—have a clear opportunity to succeed in life.

The stratification between the more affluent and those who live near or below the poverty line is persistent and clearly poses an economic problem for the United States. Schools and education can be part of the solution to create better connections to "self-actualization" to self, home, community, and in society. Reforms instituted under the No Child Left Behind Act (NCLB) have done little to bolster the country's competitiveness in preparing our youth for the future. Frauenheim and Yamamoto (2009) contend "that the root of the issue has always remained within the U. S. borders, in an institution not often mentioned in today's political rhetoric: the classroom" (n.p.).

This chapter explores the relationships of income potential to health and education. According to a study done by the nonprofit "Education Trust" in 2002, an estimated 2.4 million dropouts between the ages 16 and 24 end up jobless, and the numbers are growing. Many of these students come from areas where education is present but with few resources and less-qualified teachers than found in wealthier areas.

Education provides opportunities for individuals to seek their level of interest and potential. But by demanding results without readiness to learn from all corners of society, the 2.4 million-plus continue to fail. Education completion is but one indicator for our nation to continue to develop and prosper. We are part of an international society and must be prepared to participate at a high level. Our children need real reform in schooling to be prepared for a future that is fast moving and ever changing.

To bring improved growth to US society, Frauenheim and Yamamoto (2009) explain, "The key to the school's approach is not training students in a particular skill that could soon be obsolete, but rather develop critical thinking and project management" (n.p.).

Where better to start than at the preschool level with hands-on exploration and problem solving? Why not have children use engineering practices in building, problem-solving projects that involve discovery and cooperation? Motivation and accomplishment come from success at an early age, not from paper and pencil drills at ages when children are developmentally not ready.

If education does not become more relevant to future needs and opportunity, high school dropout rates will continue to increase and enrollment in postsecondary education will decrease. Minorities and those with little wealth, while growing in population, are either dropping out before completing high school or declining in enrollments at colleges and universities. And enrollment of white males in colleges has steadily declined over the last decade.

Mulvey (2009) writes: "America's boys are being left behind by current practices in the classroom. Statistically, they are performing less well than they were 10 years ago. Boys are dropping out of high schools in significant numbers, failing to complete college degrees and behaving more violently" (p. 34).

School practices, family involvement, preventative health care and early readiness are part of the solution to success and motivation for learning. But schools must drastically reform their curricula to a relevant material and practical implementation. Each of the former criteria is essential for educating a future society that is healthy and prosperous.

Housing Values and Education Quality

Economists strive to build models to show that quality of local education has a persistent effect on quality and costs of local homes. In 2010, Chiodo, Hernández-Murillo, and Owyang for the Federal Reserve Bank analyzed the housing values and school district achievement measures in the St. Louis metropolitan area and explained these relationships:

> We reexamine the relationship between quality of public schools and house prices and find it to be nonlinear. Unlike most studies in the literature, we determined that the price premium parents must pay to buy a house in an area associated with a better school increases as school quality increases. This is true even after controlling for neighborhood characteristics, such as the racial composition of neighborhoods, which is also capitalized into house prices. (2010, pp. 185–186)

Interesting to see that the economics of house costs, based on school quality, overcomes the former issue of whether a white family, for example, would buy a house in a neighborhood of African American owners. It appears so—if the schools for their children are good.

But, of course, the relationships intersect in complex ways, as families with higher incomes can afford to buy (or rent) a fancier, more expensive house or apartment, one usually located in a district with better schools. So better schools can help to drive up housing prices; and then better schools will attract families who can and do pay higher property taxes that help school funding. These parents often demand higher performance from their children's schools—and from their children ("*Turn Off the tv and Do Your Homework!!*"). Intersecting goes all ways: that is, better homes sell for higher prices, that are consumed by richer buyers, who fund (taxes and contributions), and expect better schools—and the cycle rolls on!

Education and Income

The level of education and/or training parallels the later income and wealth of the individual. As shown in Chapter 6, each step on the

Table 10.1   Lifetime Earnings Variations within Education Levels, 2009 Dollars

Education Levels	25th Percentile $	75th Percentile $	Interquartile Range $
Less than High School	$ 644,600	$ 1,464,000	$ 819,400
High School Diploma	867,500	1,889,500	1,022,000
Some College/No Degree	1,035,500	2,252,100	1,216,700
Associate's Degree	1,177,100	2,426,300	1,249,200
Bachelor's Degree	1,490,600	3,388,700	1,898,100
Master's Degree	1,864,400	3,835,600	1,971,200
Doctoral Degree	2,150,400	4,743,400	2,592,900
Professional Degree	2,004,600	6,472,800	4,468,200

Source: Anthony P. Carnevale, Stephen J. Rose, and Ban Cheah (2009).

education ladder increases the likelihood of greater earning power. Not only does the power of earning increase but the choice of profession is also advanced. So while a PhD at a college or university may not have the same wage potential as a BA in business or commerce, the choice for a profession is opportune and satisfying.

Statistics estimate the difference of approximately 838 dollars monthly between the PhD and no college in wage pay but does not take into account job satisfaction that is statistically even greater.

Table 10.1 compares the ranges of income by education for those at the lower and upper percentiles and the difference "inter-quartile range" in 2009. The range is tremendous, between the lowest 25th percentile for high school dropouts at $644,600 over a lifetime, or at $1,464,000 in the 75th percentile of dropouts, and those with a professional degree who earn, on average $2.005 million in the 25th and $6.472 million in the 75th percentile, over a lifetime. Thus, not only does per-week pay rise with education, but also lifetime earnings show even greater differences by education attainment and level. And even the ages of the family when they start having children is changing.

Starting Families Later and Earlier

Society is changing and aging. Not only are people living longer, they are putting off marriage, childbirth, and parenting until their 30s and 40s. The exception to this is in our inner cities where teenage pregnancy is on the rise. Both situations cause a heavy burden on our education system: first, later parenting patterns involve career-minded mothers who return to work soon after birth, and second, early teenage pregnancy occuring too often without a supporting spouse.

In both scenarios, the school system is burdened with either after school care for the career family or a need for early child education programs to develop readiness skills for children born to young and inexperienced women. According to the Guttmacher Institute (2010), "For the first time since the early 1990's, overall rates of pregnancy and birth—among teenagers and young women increased from 2005 to 2006. Preliminary data on births for 2007 show a further increase among all women including teenagers" (p. 4).

Further research indicates that women who are educated and working in career tracks are putting off childbearing until later in life. The increase in teenage pregnancy remains prevalent in poor and minority groups exacerbating the issue of healthy childcare and preparation for schooling.

And according to an article in the *New England Journal of Medicine* (2005), there have been major demographic shifts in childbearing for older women in the United States. "The number of first births per 1,000 women from 35 to 39 years of age increased by 36 percent between 1991 and 2001, and the rate among women 40 to 44 years of age increased by a remarkable 70 percent" (p. 18).

As jobs become more specialized and technological, some youth remain in school longer, seeking to learn a skill needed in the workplace. These are the students who delay marriage or partnerships, child rearing, and home responsibilities. In addition, they produce one or two children but are stable economically and contribute to the commonwealth of the country. Students who are raised and schooled in or near the poverty level, often dropout, have several children, and often have to rely on their families or public assistance for sustenance contributing little or nothing to the wealth of the nation. As low-skilled jobs disappear, so do the opportunities for those unschooled or untrained.

Our nation must open our eyes to the importance of early education, training those who have been disenfranchised by the current system and assessing skills of all its populace so that we can prosper as individuals and as a nation.

Good Schools are Essential

As income increases, the chance of finding housing within a highly rated school system increases, and a child's chance of success follows suit. As income decreases, opportunities for schools become less desirable with fewer resources and less chance of academic success.

Communities are formed with similar interests, prospects, and expectations. People seek housing to suit their pocket first, but those with greater understanding and enriched background also prefer good public or private schools. Those who are on the lower socioeconomic scale seek housing for basic needs of shelter and cannot afford to think much of how schools may affect their child's future.

While those with more wealth rely on real estate agents to find the correct neighborhoods with all their criteria. Those with no wealth seek housing simply according to their ability to pay or where public subsidy allows them to live. Thus, where children go to school is determined by family income and the quality of schooling follows the money.

Private School Choice. Public Schools are the mainstay of America's education system with approximately 49 million attending. However, 5.5 million children attend private schools, both religious and nonsectarian (Kraushaar, 1970). The choice of public or private rests, once more, with the income of the family and their ability to pay. These families have the option to enroll in private day or residential institutions and can also afford the special help in any area, if needed. Families who live in poor sections of cities, or desolate rural areas have to accept whatever schooling is available to them.

Charter schools have begun, with some success, to offer a better environment for schooling within poorer communities. And while families might choose the charter school, they must rely on random selection by lottery that offers no assurance that their child will be selected. The lack of equity in schooling has a huge impact on families, communities, and society. Who will pay in the long run as we neglect quality education for all of our children?

Extracurricular Advantages. Schools in wealthier districts have not had to eliminate their arts' programs. Music, band, orchestra, visual arts, painting/drawing are still an integral part of the curriculum. Students are involved in clubs from chess to engineering, where they experience valuable skills academically and aesthetically for a more enriched future. Parents with resources can select language schools or private lessons to reinforce music, dance, or other interests that their children might have.

The ability to travel, experience summer camps, and attend events at museums, theater, or cultural centers are all part of an invaluable education experience reserved for the well to do and unattainable by the poor.

Extra assistance in academic areas or in mental health is easily accessible and contracted. Parent with no means must be content with schools that have all but eliminated extracurricular activities, where the curricula is based only on state or national standards and where focus is on passing mandated tests. Extra help is required by title programs but consists of more of the same drill (to pass the tests). It is no wonder that these student quickly tire of school and lose their motivation to continue through high school or beyond.

Perhaps, if policy makers and the more affluent were required to send their children to underfunded schools, they would understand not only the present plight of the child but they would also understand the lost revenue to society.

Private Schools

While Beutow (1970, 1983) and others have analyzed the role and importance of Catholic schools in American education history, less research has looked at the changing mix of private and parochial schools, and whether these schools are growing or not. If families are to have access to a range of school choices locally, the parents will need both *resources* to help pay for this education and *choices* of schools to send their children.

American Catholic schools had long provided available, inexpensive, or free options for poor (often immigrant) family; now, however, the numbers dropped from a peak of over 13,000 Catholic schools to nearly half as much, at under 7,000 schools (Youniss and Convey, 2004).

Meanwhile, other types of private schools that are not Catholic have grown, including Lutheran, Methodist, Jewish, Islamic, and nonsectarian schools such as Montessori, ethical culture, military academies, and independent day and boarding schools. Since the peak year for Catholic school enrollments was 1965 (McCloskey, 1969), with 5.66 million students enrolled while other private school students were around a 0.5 million (Cattaro, 2002), we see the two sectors crossing in around 1985, and the non-Catholic private schools continuing to grow while Catholic schools continue to decline.

Currently, private schools overall enroll about 6 million students that include "homeschool children" as well. The non-Catholic school enrollments number almost 4 million, while Catholic school student numbers are down to over 2 million. Thus, it has become more expensive, without vouchers or charter status, for poor families to afford a nonpublic school alternative.

Unfortunately, the downward trend in the Catholic school sector appears to be continuing (Cooper, 2008). But we do see other private schools filling some of void, although many are too costly for poorer families. Charter schools are helpful, and five states now have "voucher" programs, that give parents funds (in the form of a certificate) that they can "cash in" at a nearby private school, if they can gain entrance (Lawrence, 2004).

Catholic schools historically (Bryk, Lee, and Holland, 1993) afforded a private education to those who were not able to access more expensive private institutions, but who wanted a better education than what the public schools could provide. Inner-city children were subsidized by parishes and dioceses to attend schools that were more structured and disciplined in their implementation. In a study by Coleman, Kilgore, and Hoffer (1982), the performance of parochial schools showed achievement levels above comparable public schools in the same neighborhoods.

So we do see some "privatization" of education, even in Catholic charter schools (see Weinberg, 2002). Public schools in Washington, DC, are in competition with the charter system as parents hope to be able to win the lottery, the charter lottery that is, so that their children can reap the promise of a sound education. Chicago and other large cities cannot supply the demand for charter school choice (Nelson, 2008).

Timothy F. C. Knowles, head of the Urban Education Institute in Chicago states, "there's a very high demand for our schools...we are turning away three of four people for every slot" (Haederle, 2011).

In Washington, DC, for example, the public schools are declining while charter schools are taking their place. Since charter schools are usually run by private individuals or agencies, but are fully funded by the government, they stand between the two sectors, offering choice and autonomy associated with private education, but funds and support provided by the public sector (Cooper, 2010).

The latest Washington, DC, data show that enrollment in charter schools jumped 9 percent to 32,009, while regular DC public schools also grew, but much less at 1 percent to 46,191 after years of decline. Thus, today the nation's capital has the largest percentage of students in charter schools, meaning that more families are staying in the system, and using either a public school, or a publicly supported "private" one—a bringing together of public resources and private choice, as Cooper explains (2010):

> A "golden mean" should mean the best of both worlds, not two educational worlds in conflict, as has been the case during recent decades. The United States has a long and noble tradition of endeavoring to educate every child at the highest possible level, regardless of race, color, ethnicity, creed, or geographic location. At the same time, Americans have always been and remain a deeply religious people, with 65 percent professing a belief in God, the highest in the modern world (see also, Mulvey, Cooper, and Maloney, 2010).

Mayor Antonio Villaraigosa of Los Angeles put the word out to charter schools, to help the public schools and the community—bringing together private initiative, public funds, and local children under one roof, another example of the intersecting going on in cities and their schools. In the mayor's words:

> We must start blurring the lines between charter and traditional schools until the distinctions cease to exist. And we need to end once and for all the damaging us-versus-them mentality that has polluted relations between school districts and the charter community and jeopardized the potential for meaningful reform and positive change that benefits all students. Imagine a public school system that creates a true variety of good choices, rather than a behemoth of a bureaucracy that centrally governs our schools. (Ravitch, 2010, p. 11)

School Restructuring. While the United States has expanded its precollege and college courses for the middle and upper classes, the vocational and career training programs have disappeared, meaning that the less academic and poorer kids have fewer options and face a difficult time after leaving schools in finding jobs and making a living.

The lower tuition, ranging (from $1,900 to $2,300 per year), created an opportunity for families, many of whom were not Catholic, to select a private school within their means and to better the education of their children, who otherwise might attend inner city, low performing schools (Nelson, 1998).

Charter schools are beginning to have an impact on some of the poorer kids, especially in inner cities. Parents must be aware of the difference between their current public school and the offerings of a local charter school. But even if they choose the charter option, they must enter a lottery to gain admission. So once again, even if poor parents want a better choice for their child, it is simply left to chance with no alternative if their name is not pulled (see Weinberg, 2002).

Educational Impact on the Nation

Several variables influence students' attending, completing, and going beyond the K-12 system. Beginning with a healthy childhood, early readiness for a rigorous curriculum, subsidized programs for those unable to afford a quality preschool program and scientific-research-based learning. If put in place, we see the possibility of a more educated populace and a society rich in economic independence.

The *Christian Science Monitor* reports that the United States is making some progress on its high school graduation rate, with an increase of 3.5 percent over the years from 2002 to 2009. The graduation percentage nationwide has increased from 72 to 75 percent; but 40 percent of minorities still fail to graduate or finish high school. Some states have made better progress than others; for example, New York and Tennessee have shown the largest gains, while Arizona, California, and others fail to graduate even 60 percent of their students.

Graduation rates, as reported by states, must be looked at carefully as they often do not reflect how many students dropped out prior to their senior year. Perhaps an even more telling statistic is the US placement on the PISA (Program for International Student Assessment) in 2010. Ranked seventeenth in Reading, thirty-first in Mathematics, and twenty-second in Science, it is clear that our present programs and student engagement are lacking somewhere.

The nonprofit education trust cautions that dropout rates result in high unemployment and the number is rising. According to Frauenheim and Yamamoto (2009), "About 2.4 million dropouts between the ages of 16–24 were unemployed last year, 9 percent more than two years previously... And the problem may be even worse, because states inflate their graduation numbers... sometimes by 30 percent" (n.p.).

There should be a renewed effort to improve education by attending to families, the young, and curricula for all students.

College Completion. College completion in the United States has been declining over the last several decades. While once a world leader, the United States is now twelfth among 36 developed countries (Lewin, 2010). In a *New York Times* article, Gaston Caperton, president of the College Board announced, "The growing education deficit is no less a threat to our nations well-being than the current fiscal crisis" (p. A11).

Minorities and low-income students suffer a worse result with only 30 percent of African American and 20 percent of Latino youth earning any postsecondary degrees. This poses a problem for our nation as jobs require training and/or higher education for student to become self-sufficient. The College Board made five recommendations to remediate the current crisis:

1. state-financed pre-school program
2. better high school and middle school counseling
3. dropout prevention programs
4. alignment with international curricular standards
5. improved teacher quality. (*New York Times,* see Lewin, July 23, 2010, p. A11)

Education Benefits

The benefits of higher education are threefold; first, it gives individuals a choice of career and employment; second it contributes to the wealth of our nation; and third, higher education contributes to society as a whole. Thus, higher earnings, choice of career, and contribution to society should be motivators to reform our education system to meet the higher education goal. Disparities and inequities in funding for schools result in missed opportunities for all persons to contribute to their own well-being and to the society. Baum and Payea (2005) contend, "Education does pay... it has a high rate of return for student from all racial/ethnic groups, for men, women, for those from all family backgrounds" (p. 6).

An educated populace is healthier, contributing more to tax revenues, enjoying a better quality of life, and enhancing and participating in a strong democratic society. Family life is improved through education. Without the stress of having to provide only essentials, families can enjoy activities together, help and reinforce students' homework, and experience cultural events that further enhance learning and happiness.

Baum and Payea (2005) further state, "In addition to increasing material standards of living, reduced poverty improves the overall well being of society... individuals are more likely to engage in organized volunteer work, to vote, donate blood... and less likely to be incarcerated" (p. 9).

As Americans stay in school longer, and complete degrees, or vocational training, the nation enjoys a return from their experience. All workers, in the professional or vocational fields, benefit from the collaborative and productive work of their colleagues and peers. Thus, education is the key to a healthy society: prosperity, healthy lifestyles, family stability, contributions and volunteer work, collaboration, and participation in the democratic process.

Limitations on Women

In general, the better the education, the higher the income. That's in general. In particular, however, education alone may not be enough. We know that even when women are well-prepared and educated, they may have problems competing for the jobs and the top positions in the world of work. This limit, that is the "glass ceiling," is particularly acute for women, even though they are gaining on men in their education and the workplace.

Traditionally, going back 30 years, women still earned less than men, even with the same or better education attainment and degrees. As explained earlier, men on average earn $2 million more than women over their work lives (US Bureau of Labor Statistics, 2004). Even a high school diploma makes a differences in annual income, ranging from $340,000 to $800,000 for men, while women make less. And the opportunities to attend college are large and lead to better jobs, more income, and the opportunities better to raise and support a family.

And attending college seems to be more critical now in the modern, high technological competitive era than ever before. Here are some reasons that an education in college is so important:

Greater Job Opportunities. We know from data over the years that a college degree helps to increase the job chances and choices, while giving the family greater flexibility and mobility. While women are beginning to catch up, and are for first time earning more than men coming out of college in some regions, the differences still prevail for women of color and are worse for men of color (Levin et al., 2007).

This is not to say that skilled craftsmen and artists are not still also on demand. We shall always want quality people to build our homes, fix our plumbing, and keep our computers running well. So the interconnection between good jobs, income, and past and future education remain strong and important.

More Income. The long-term impact of education is enormous, so an investment in education remains critical to the family and the society. We need ways of making college more accessible, longer, and cheaper. Why can't seniors in high schools take college credit courses in math, science, and English, instead of wasting their twelfth grade year with filler courses, and useless "electives?" The payoff's are clear and have been for a long time.

Regular Jobs and More Job Options. In changing and diminishing job markets, we know that education provides greater insurance of keeping a job, and/or finding a new one. Educated workers often have greater access, and can adapt their skills and experience to new and changing markets and needs.

Flexibility and Marketability in Work and Careers. So many students complete high school and go into college without learning a skill or applying their talents. More and more education means preparing for life, in a flexible manner, where learning skills and a work ethic can give options and make adults more marketable (Longley, 2009). It all comes together: better schooling, better health, better jobs, and the social skills to do well in the community and in the job.

Life Skill Building. Overall, education in school, starting early, prepares students for life: living and working together with others, ethical behavior, and responsibility. The interconnections are never clearer: better social preparation, stronger and more flexible job skills, and enhanced relations to community, increased income, better schooling for offspring, and access to good health care from prenatal through life. Education thus builds both "social capital" within the family and community and "human capital" in the society and the workplace (Romboy, 2000).

Conclusion

This chapter has traced the importance of starting education early, and continuing through life. Children from middle- and upper-class families have playgroups and prekindergarten programs, often allowing their parents to work, at least part-time, and for the children to benefit from the opportunities. We have seen the differences between those who can afford a good school—either private or in a good neighborhood—and it effects on health, learning, and future income.

Understanding the characteristics of ethnic/racial groups, their background, early educational support, family aspirations, and community values can make the difference in whether students leave school prematurely or continue on to postsecondary education.

Kuh, Kinzie, Buckley, Bridges, and Hayek (2006) list the following six key precollege experiences for all students to gain access and to succeed in life (p. 17). These six include the following: (1) family and peer support, (2) demographic characteristics, including race, gender, and SES, (3) motivation to learn, (4) academic preparation, (5) aptitude and college readiness, and (6) enrollment choices.

The United States must recognize the essentials for quality education for all its citizens—starting earlier and extending longer—if we want to close the achievement gap and remain in a leadership position internationally. Middle-class families have long enrolled their children in preschools and playgroups; now all children should have these opportunities.

As Stegelin (2004) explained "how quality early childhood education has the greatest positive effect on children from lower socioeconomic status, children who are at-risk, because of other circumstances, and children with disabilities and special needs" (p. 116).

References

Baum, S., and Payea, K. (2005). *The benefits of higher education for individuals and society.*

Bryk, A. S., Lee, V. E., & Holland, P. B. (1993). *Catholic schools and the common good.* Cambridge, MA: Harvard University Press.

Buetow, H. A. (1983). *A history of Catholic schools and the common good.* Washington, DC: National Catholic Education Association.

———. (1970). *Of singular benefit: The story of Catholic education in the U.S.* Washington, DC: National Catholic Education Association.

Carnevale, A. P., Rose, S. J., & Cheah, B. (2009). *The college payoff: Education, occupations and life-time earnings.* Washington, DC: Georgetown University Center on Education and the Workforce.

Cattaro, G. M. (2002). Immigration and pluralism in urban Catholic schools. *Education and Urban Society, 34*(2), 199–211.

Chiodo, A. J., Hernández-Murillo, R., & Owyang, M. T. (2010, May/June). Nonlinear effects of school quality on house prices. *Review of the Federal Reserve Bank of St. Louis, 92*(3), 185–204.

Coleman, J. S., Hoffer, T., & Kilgore, S. (1982). *High school achievement: Public, Catholic, and privates schools compared.* New York: Basic Books.

College Board. Retrieved from www.collegeboard.com/prod_downloads/_EducationPays2004pdf.

Cooper, B. S. (2010, October 10). Commentary: Public, private school convergence presents policy opportunities. *School Reform News.* Center for School Reform, Heartland Institute.

———. (2008). Foreword, to *Religious charter schools: Legalities and practicalities,* by Lawrence D. Weinberg. Charlotte, NC: Information Age Publishing, iii–vii.

Cooper, B. S., McSween, R. B. & Murphy, T. (2012). Finding a golden mean in education policy: Centering religious and private schools. *Peabody Journal of Education* 83(2) 20–29.

Frauenheim, E., & Yamamoto, M. (2009). Offshoring: U. S. needs reforms not rhetoric. *CNET* Retrieved from cnetnews.com2009–1070_5198156htm.

Furstenberg, F. F. (2010, Spring). On a new schedule: Transitions to adulthood and Family change. *Transitions to Adulthood. 20*(1), 43–51.

Greeley, A. M. (1967). *The Catholic experience: An interpretation of the history of American Catholicism.* Garden City, NY: Doubleday & Co.

Griffee, S. L., & Schulten, K. (2011, September 29). College graduation rates stagnate. *New York Times,* Education, 4.

Guttmacher Institute (2010, January). *U. S. teenage pregnancies, births, abortions: National and state trends and trends by race and ethnicity.*

Haederle, M. (2011). *Chicago charter schools aim to lift urban education.* Pacific Standard. Retrieved from www.psmag.com/ education/Chicago-charter-schools-aim-to-lift-urban-education-34328.

Kraushaar, O. F. (1970). *American nonpublic schools: Patterns in diversity.* Baltimore, MD: Johns Hopkins University Press.

Kuh, G. D., Kinze, J., Buckley, J., Bridges, B. K., & Hayek, J. C. (2006, July) *What matters to student success: A review of the literature.* Commissioned Report for the National Symposium on Postsecondary Student Success: Spearheading a Dialog on Student Success.

Lawrence, S. (2004). "New" immigrants in the Catholic schools: A preliminary assessment. In J. Youniss & J. J. Convey (Eds.), *Catholic schools at the crossroads: Survival and transformation* (pp. 178–200). New York: Teachers College Press.

Levin, H. M., Belfield, C., Muennig, P., & Roused, C. (2007). The public returns to public educational investments in African-American males. *Economics of Education Review, 26,* 700–709.

Lewin, T. (2010, July 23). Once a leader, U.S. lags in college degrees. Education, *New York Times,* p. A11.

Longley, R. (2009). *Lifetime earnings soar with education.* Retrieved from usgov-info.about.com/od/moneymatters/a/edandearnings.htm.

McCloskey, N. J. (1969). *Catholic education faces its future.* Garden City, NY: Double Day.

McDonald, D. (2005). United States Catholic elementary and secondary schools 2004–2005. *The Annual Statistical Report on Schools, Enrollment and Staff.* Washington, DC: National Catholic Educational Association.

Mulvey, J. D. (2009). Feminization of schools: What it is doing to our boys. *The School Administrator.* September 2009.

Mulvey, J. D., Cooper, B. S., & Maloney, A. S. (2010). *Blurring the lines: Charter, public, private and religious schools coming together.* Charlotte, NC: Information Age Publishing.

Nelson, M. S. (1998). Catholic elementary schools in Chicago's black inner city: Four modes of adaptation to environmental changes. *Nonprofit and Voluntary Sector Quarterly, 23*(3), 209–225.

———. (2000). Black Catholic schools in inner-city Chicago: Forging a path to the future. In James Youniss & John J. Convey (Eds.) *Catholic schools at the crossroads: Survival and transformation* (pp. 157–177). New York: Teachers College Press.

Morris, R. (2005, November 4). Delaying childbearing: How old is too old? *New England journal of Medicine* p. 1. www.pregnancyandbaby.com

Ravitch, D. (2010, March 14). The push back on charter schools: Opinion pages, *New York Times,* p. A–9.

Romboy, D. (2000, July 11). Human capital called key to U.S. success in Information Age. *Deseret New,* D6 & D8.

Stegelin, D. (2004). Early childhood education. In F. P. Schargel & J. Smink (Eds). *Helping students graduate: A strategic approach to dropout prevention* (pp. 115–123). Larchmont, NY: Eye on Education.

Weinberg, L. (2002). The constitutionality of religion-based charter schools: Answering the practical legal questions (2004). Dissertation completed at Boston University, College of Education.

Youniss, J., & Convey, J. J. (Eds.) (2004). *Catholic schools at the crossroads: Survival and transformation.* New York: Teachers College Press.

11

Can "Separate But Equal" Schools Work?

Introduction

This chapter focuses on the despair and hope for public education in the United States. As we have become more segregated and in some quarters more intolerant, it is time to look at our future as a country: a country that has been and is made up of diversity. Demographic changes are on the horizon, as the once-dominant culture is becoming the minority; and we, as a whole society, must make sure that those who become the majority are educated, healthy, and wise.

Today, the vestiges of discrimination have restrengthened, in schools, in neighborhoods, and in society. Gary Orfield (2009) writes, "Schools in the United States are more segregated today than they have been in four decades" (p. 11). Sadly, the work done by reformers and progressives, dating back before the 1954 *Brown* decision, has been undone by the Robert's court in 2007.

A Brief History of Desegregation

A brief review of the historical battles to equalize education for all children is important to understand, as we attempt to bring about real change in a demographically shifting society. Racial segregation was outlawed and discouraged in the 1950s with court cases; but today, we see resegregation in urban, suburban, and rural communities. This section compares what's happening now, reversing the *Brown* ruling, which is causing more separation and less equality in our schools and society. First, we review *Brown,* and its fascinating language and intent, followed by events and developments that separate us, not only by race and language, but also by income and wealth.

The US Supreme Court, in 1954, decided:

Segregation of children in the public schools solely on the basis of race denies to black children the equal protection of the laws guaranteed under the Fourteenth Amendment, even though the physical facilities and other may be equal. Education in public schools is a right, which must be made available to all on equal terms.

And Chief Justice Earl Warren continued:

Separating black children from others solely because of their race generates a feeling of inferiority as to their status in the community that may affect their hearts and minds in a way unlikely ever to be undone. The impact of segregation is greater when it has the sanction of law. A sense of inferiority affects the motivation of a child to learn.

Segregation with the sanction of law tends to impede the educational and mental development of black children and deprives them of some of the benefits they would receive in an integrated school system. Whatever may have been the extent of psychological knowledge at the time of *Plessy v. Ferguson*, modern authority amply supports this finding. Thus, any language to the contrary in *Plessy v. Ferguson* is rejected. (*Brown v. Board of Education*, 349 US 294, 1955)

The result did not guarantee cooperation or compliance; many riots, protests, and arguments continued by the white majority, and minority children were confronted with abject discrimination. On the positive side, many communities began to embrace racial diversity, seeing it as a natural and enriching experience for all students. Today, as the country becomes even more diverse, learning, working, and socializing together must be seen as strength for democracy, the economy, and stability.

But although the *Brown* ruling by the Supreme Court that separate children by race in schools were inherently unequal, racial and ethnic segregation continues in every state of our nation. The percentage of black students in 90–100 percent minority schools grew from 33.9 percent in 1992 to 45 percent in 1997; the percentage of Hispanic students in these schools was up from 28 percent to 35.4 percent in 1997 (Orfield and Yun, 1999). Segregated by neighborhoods and socioeconomic status, many schools have taken on the character of poverty and in turn have become representative of the original separate and unequal problem.

Supreme Court Judge John Roberts (June 28, 2007) reinforced the separate and unequal standing when it ruled that race alone could not determine whether schools can be integrated, thus overturning, the intent of the *Brown* decision. In his dissent to the ruling, however, Justice John Paul Stevens (2007) responded:

> There is a cruel irony in The Chief Justice's reliance on our decision in *Brown v. Board of Education*, 349 U. S. 294 (1955). The first sentence in the concluding paragraph of his opinion states: "Before *Brown*, schoolchildren were told where they could and could not go to school based on the color of their skin." This sentence reminds me of Anatole France's observation: "[T]he majestic equality of the la[w], forbid[s] rich and poor alike to sleep under bridges, to beg in the streets, and to steal their bread." The Chief Justice fails to note that it was only black schoolchildren who were so ordered; indeed, the history books do not tell stories of white children struggling to attend black schools. In this and other ways, The Chief Justice rewrites the history of one of this Court's most important decisions.

Segregation Today

A recent article in the *New York Times* by Sam Dillon (November 5, 2011) reinforces a fear that minority populations, merged into predominantly white districts, will weaken educational programs and achievement. The merger of two different districts in Tennessee—the city of Memphis and Shelby County, each with distinct demographics, black and white—has caused a firestorm, politically and socially. A former principal of a predominantly white school, now on a combined 23-member board, exploring the merger, explains, "There's the same element of fear. In the 1970s, it was a physical, personal fear. Today the fear is about the academic decline of the Shelby Schools...As far as racial trust goes...I don't think we've improved much since the 1970s" (p. 6).

The opposition to the merger is both racial and economic. Lacking in equity in school funding, teacher quality, class size, and resources, minority schools have been subject to lower investment with poorer academic results. Problems and resentment arise when funding is allocated by property wealth; according to the article, median income for families in Memphis is $32,000 while the suburban average is $92,000.

Racial disparities and numbers in the two districts fuel the anger and distrust on both sides of the issue: Memphis has 103,000 total students, and 47, 000 in Shelby—with 85 percent black and 62 percent white respectively. Achievement rates between the two districts exemplify any area where students are segregated by race and socioeconomic differences. Memphis city schools are reported as one of the lowest-scoring districts in reading and math (25.89 percent proficiency reading and

22.63 percent in math), while the more middle-class Shelby County system records 57.4 percent proficiency in reading and 48.8 percent in math.

Demographics Shift

As census data has shown, the white population in the United States will become the minority by 2040, 12 years earlier than first projected. The stability of the country—nationally and internationally—depends on quality education, productivity, and social integration. White dominance will quickly become history as the now-minority population finds voice politically, educationally, and economically. Today's education census shows a distinct gap in college completion for blacks and Hispanics.

Table 11.1 is an indicator of college completions by ethnicity and gender ages 22–28.

And data collected by Aud et al. (2010), including social inequality looked at college completion rates relative to income levels and tuition rates, show similar trends from 1996 to 2008. Young adults in this category did not earn a high school diploma, or receive some alternative credits, such as the GED.

Table 11.1   Percent College Graduation by Gender and Ethnicity, 1940–2007

Year	% college completion	
	White Non-Hispanic Male	White Non-Hispanic Female
1940	5%	3%
1980	22%	19%
1990	22%	24%
2000	24%	31%
2005–2007	24%	34%

Year	% college completion	
	Black Non-Hispanic Male	Black Non-Hispanic Female
1940	–1%	–2%
1980	9%	10.5%
1990	8.5%	11%
2000	10%	15%
2005–2007	–7 11%	17%

Source: US Census IPUMS 1980–2005–0 ACS In McDaniel, et al., Ohio State University.

Educational attainment is an absolute for earning prowess in adulthood. And earning power adds to the health and prosperity of the individual and his/her contribution to society's well-being.

If, as touted by all experts in the field of education, social workers, and neurophysicists, education is the great leveler in social mobility, why are we still in the throes of underachievement among the poor? The unfair advantages of children who attend schools with abundant resources, smaller class sizes, and more experienced teachers go unrecognized by law and policy makers in government—locally, statewide, and nationally. Equity in funding, support, and care needs to become the priority for all the underserved population. Why should a child born into poverty be condemned to impoverishment in school? The promise of "No Child Left Behind" must become a literal fact if we are to grow from within.

High-Poverty Schools

According to the National Center for Educational Statistics (May 2010), the number of high-poverty schools continues to grow in the public sector. In 2007–2008, of 196, 122 schools were identified as high poverty, an increase of 12 percent from 1999–2000 to 17 percent in 2008 (p. 5).

The indicator of free and reduced lunch for eighth grade achievement levels in reading and math show that the percentage of students in more-impoverished schools with 70–100 percent free and reduced lunch continues to score far below those with much lower percentages of free-lunch students. Poverty runs parallel to underachievement in schools as does poor health, attendance, and social ills such as incarceration and mental disease.

The stark comparison is indicative of poverty's influence in academic achievement effecting entire accomplishments throughout a lifetime. Another indicator for poor achievement is the lack of language skills necessary to pass standardized achievement tests that are used to measure proficiency. According to the National Center for Educational Statistics, the proportion of students who attend schools and have difficulty with English has increased from 10 percent in 1980 to 21 percent in 2009. Since more students lack language skills, linked with poor health and welfare, it is no wonder we are growing less efficient and less productive as a nation.

As minority cultures begin to become the majority, belief systems that originate within a segregated community need to be understood. Our expectations for others to succeed and lead must develop through greater multicultural understandings and acceptance. Although we proclaim diversity within our schools, the foundation remains based in the middle-class white cast. We can no longer ignore the statistics that show low-income, mostly minority, students as underachievers. According to National Center for Statistics,

- 47 percent of low-income students enroll in postsecondary education or trade school versus 82 percent of high-income students;
- 18 percent African American and 19 percent of Hispanic high school students earn a bachelor's degree compared to 35 percent of white students; and
- 22 percent of academically qualified low-income students do not pursue postsecondary education versus 4 percent of high-income academically qualified students.

The time for real change and reform is now, before it is too late.

Improved Schools, Improved Parental Involvement, Improved Success, and a Secure Future

No question that those who grow up and live in high-poverty areas suffer the consequences of lower academic achievement, poor medical care, and substandard housing. Schools have always served as the hope-for institution to break the cycle of poverty and improve social growth and success. The message in schools is that the more education and knowledge, the better chance for a fuller, healthier, and happier life. Yet, many high-needs public schools seem to be unable to provide the education necessary for the desired outcomes. What can schools do to change to education for children from poor neighborhoods? What are some effective and proven strategies that work well in minority and diverse school cultures?

Reformers often look to more rigid curricula, higher standards and expectations, uniform methods, and a "no excuses" approach as their mantra for success. And several schools have touted higher test scores as evidence for their accomplishments. In a recent *New York Times* report, Diane Ravitch pointed out that schools that have been designated as "success stories" are "less spectacular then they appear" (Ravitch, 2011, p. 1). While graduation rates from high schools can increase, the actual proficiency levels of the students is far below levels of acceptance.

The growth in achievement of students at the Bruce Randolph School, for example, shows that ninth grade writing scores had doubled since 2007, from 7 percent to 15 percent proficiency. Perhaps the acceptance of what works can be best described by Jonathan Alter, columnist for

Bloomberg View: "'The Bruce Randolph school should not be compared to other Colorado schools in affluent neighborhoods'; to consider Randolph's scores alongside those of white, middle-class schools was like comparing apples to oranges" (p. 1).

Common attitudes and beliefs among many of the educated white and middle class that blame students, communities, and their families for lack of substantial growth in achievement are barriers to the possibility of real reform. Celebrating a 15 percent improvement rate means that we ignore 85 percent of students who did not pass. We see successes for some students who attend poorly resourced schools. Why? What makes the difference?

Harlem Children's Zone—Promise Academies

The Harlem Children's Zone instituted a neighborhood program that included social services, health clinics, and a charter school for low-income families within a 100-block radius. The community-based program offers early childhood programs, parenting classes, job-related training centers, counseling, along with health and fitness for all residents within the designated area.

In a study of the Promise Academy operated by the Harlem Children's Zone, success has been documented by assessments in both mathematics and literacy. Researchers Roland Fryer and Will Dobbie compared student outcomes to students in New York City as a whole and to students who had entered the lottery to get into the school.

Findings from their research indicated substantial gains from sixth to eighth grade; math went from 39th percentile in sixth grade to 74th percentile in the eighth. In English language arts, percentile gains went from 39th to 53rd (Brooks, 2007).

The gains were substantial enough (1.3 and 1.4 standard deviations) such that data from this report, show that achievement gaps in these two areas "eliminated the achievement gap between its black students and the city average for white students" (Fryer, in Brooks, 2007). The Children's Zone is a complete neighborhood program that provides health and psychological services to a 100-block community, whether children are attending the school or not. Reformers agree that broader issues that afflict a community must be identified and remediated along with in-school program enhancements. For example, schools remain open after class hours creating programs for students, both remedial and recreational.

Many agree that while cultural differences should be recognized and validated, a no-nonsense approach to behavior and for responsibility must be inculcated. The theory behind the no-nonsense model stems from the role modeling often present in middle-class homes and school but too often missing in poor neighborhoods and homes. The Children's Zone has established a "no excuses" mantra for behaviors in and out of school and personal responsibility for class and homework. Assessments are an ongoing practice to determine curricula stress points and individual performance.

The Brookings Institution conducted a follow-up study to reanalyze and measure the effectiveness of the Harlem Children's Zone comparable to other New York City charter schools. In a "New Analysis," Whitehurst and Croft (2010) refute some of the findings of Fryer and Dobbie, comparing outcomes of the Harlem Promise Academy with other charter schools, and examining the cost effectiveness of neighborhood social service networks. In their analysis they pose, "If a schools-only approach works as well or better than a schools-plus community philosophy, this finding has huge consequences for education policy, going to the heart of how public funds should be allocated to enhance educational achievement and reduce socioeconomic disparities" (p. 3).

Since a random and/or experimental approach would be unethical when dealing with minors and students, Brookings collected data on the outcomes on tests and performances at other charter schools in the city. Using a school-only-based approach, they found that other charter schools representing the same demographic performed as well or better than the Promise Academy.

Thus, the question posed by the Brookings Institution was, "Does the Children's Zone produce exceptional academic achievement? If it does, that is an opportunity for Promise Neighborhoods. If it doesn't, it isn't."

The initial analysis conducted by the Booking's Institution compared state assessment scores in Math and English language arts between the Harlem Promise Academy and an average of 14 other charter schools in Manhattan and the Bronx. Data for assessment scores were based on the exact grades and standardized assessments:

2007: Grades 6, 7, and 8
2008: Grades 3, 7, and 8
2009: Grades 3, 4, 5, and 8.

Two of the Harlem Children's Zone were included in the state database comparison, The Harlem Promise Academy serving students from elementary through high school and the second Harlem Children's Academy elementary school. Findings indicate that several of the city's charter schools performed at "far superior" level to the Harlem academies, but did not indicate whether any services from community health or social services networks were provided at those sites. It should be noted, however, that the study found a ten-point difference in performance for students attending the Harlem academies in comparison to students of like demographics racially and socioeconomically attending traditional public schools.

One strong similarity between the Harlem and other city charter schools is that parents must advocate for their children, place their names for selection in a lottery, and attempt to pursue school choice for optimum results. Families who are interested in gaining a better education for their children, but cannot afford private schooling, explore alternatives with higher expectations, that their children will reach higher achievement. "Thus the enrollment in any particular school is a joint function of parental interest in that school and the school's recruiting efforts" (http://www.brooking.edu/reports/2010/0720_hcz_whitehurst.aspx).

Overall we find that the majority of charter schools in New York City have more positive test results and favorably compare to their traditional counterparts with similar demographic contour. Whitehurst and Croft (2010) affirm:

> The HCZ Promise Academy scores 10 points above its predicted score on the state assessment, which is about .6 of the school-level standard deviation for all NYC schools for grade 8 math in 2009. Thus students attending the HCZ Promise Academy are doing impressively better than students of their backgrounds attending a typical public school in NYC. (www.brooking.edu/reports/2010/0720_hczwhitehurst.aspx)

Knowledge is Power Program (KIPP) Charter Schools

KIPP schools began in 1994 and by 2008 had 50 middle-level schools with increased numbers on the elementary and high school levels. The intent of the KIPP charter schools was to serve low-socioeconomic and minority students across the nation. Praised for their work in underserved communities and higher than expected proficiency on standardized tests, KIPP schools have also come under scrutiny for harsh discipline and lack of sustainability in students' retention and test results.

The KIPP schools were the highest performing of all the charters in the study. And what the Brookings Institution study attempted to show was that quality programs, leadership, and high expectations can achieve success without the social networks represented in the Harlem Children's Zone program. KIPP's enrollment, like other charters, is determined on a lottery system. The leadership and teaching staff share school-level decision making. The tenets of their program are the more time spent in school, including days, weeks of the year, the higher the academic expectations. And with a focus on measurable results, students, parents, and teachers sign a "Commitment to Excellence" agreement.

According to KIPP's annual report card, "85 percent of KIPP students are eligible for free or reduced-price meals, 60 percent of students are African American, and 35 percent are Latino" (http://givewell.org/united_states/process/common-evaluation-problems).

What the KIPP schools fail to report are the statistics of those who drop out for poor performance along the way and are not readmitted. In a comprehensive study done by the Stanford Research Institute International (SRI International, 2008), findings indicate a major drop in enrollment by 60 percent after sixth grade. And according to the report KIPP children "experienced substantial student attrition over the same period—22 percent and 50 percent respectively…as those who leave before 8th grade have lower test scores on entering and demonstrate smaller gains" (Woodworth et al. 2008, p. 9).

Teachers and students spend 9.5 hours per day in school with large blocks of time, about 85 minutes, on both literacy and math. Retention rates depend on proficiency by fifth grade. Summer school and Sundays are also dedicated to instructional time for intervention and remedial work. An interesting analysis done by SRI indicates that those students who remain in KIPP after eighth grade entered with higher test scores initially than those with lower results. "These analyses show that a student who enters KIPP with an NCE score of 20 has a 70% chance of exiting KIPP before eighth grade, whereas a student who enters KIPP with an NCE score of 50 has a 50% chance of exiting" (Woodworth et al. 2008, p. 16).

KIPP schools have also been successful in gaining higher math scores on average when compared to similar demographics attending public schools. KIPP is a charter school that relies on parent choice and motivation for their children to learn. Results, however, are difficult to measure because of the rates of attrition and lack of sustainability of the student population.

Practices, dedication to student learning, high expectations, long hours, intervention, remedial classes, and a longer school year are all part of a reform movement to increase the overdue needs of impoverished and underserved communities. KIPP is dedicated to the hopes of poor communities, demanding hard work by students and staff. The results are certainly mixed; but questions remain as to the initial readiness for the "stayers" and "leavers" at KIPP, and whether the practices implemented would work in public schools without other service networks and help.

90/90/90 Schools—and Beyond

The 90/90/90 schools are another example of a program aimed at success for underprivileged students and communities, and was originally named from observations in Milwaukee, Wisconsin, and were founded on the following characteristics:

- More than *90 percent* of students were eligible for free or reduced lunch
- More than *90 percent* were from ethnic minority groups, and
- More than *90 percent* were meeting the district or state standards in reading or in another academic area.

The appeal of this analysis is that no one program is associated with the success of the researched schools. Inclusive of elementary through high school, data were collected on about 130,000 students in 228 different school building, including students with similar demographics from lower-socioeconomic strata. Interestingly in the study, Reeves (2003) included "student populations...ranged from schools whose populations were overwhelmingly poor and/or minority to schools that were largely Anglo and/or economically advantaged" (p. 1).

Reeves concedes that a direct link between poverty and academic failure exists; but he postulates in the schools observed that the programs initiated and the results of those programs debunk the claim that poorer students would do worse than richer ones. 90/90/90 is not a program that can be packaged and sold; it is a compilation of practices that may vary for school to school, but with commonalities (Peters and Waterman, 1982). *In Search of Excellence,* using their findings of what makes organizations excellent, Reeves et al., (2003) found five common practices similar in the 90/90/90 schools:

1. A focus on academic achievement
2. Clear curriculum choices
3. Frequent assessment of students' progress and multiple opportunities for improvement
4. An emphasis on non-fiction reading and writing, and
5. Collaborative scoring of students' work (p. 12).

The focus on student achievement takes a very different approach than the standardized tests of proficiency or not. In many schools, calculations are made on student achievement in all areas. The mantra used is: "It is not how you start here, but how you finish". Assessments were done indicating the beginning levels in students' literacy, with a focus on reading and writing for up to three hours a day, continuing until proficiency is reached. According to the individual nature of remedial needs, no one program is prescribed for all; but selections are made of interventions best suited to the needs of each student.

The belief is that focusing on the core subjects and reaching proficiency will, and does, according to Reeves (2003), translate into successes in other subjects, such as science, social studies and the arts. We agree: literacy is, in fact, the foundation for all subjects; without it, no meaning or application can be made to others areas—be they academic, or in the trades. Those who are proficient in reading, writing, and mathematics are at an advantage because they will improve their chances at better employment and social mobility.

True for most of the 90/90/90 schools, students who enter are significantly below grade level. Assessments are driven, and teachers must not use standing to label or punish students—but rather to find a starting point for each individual student to begin and progress. Written responses on tests are mandated as part assessment to create data and strategies geared to the needs of the student. According to Reeves, "The benefits of emphases on writing appear to be two-fold. First, students process information in a much clearer way...they write to 'think' and thus gain the opportunity to clarify their own thought processes" (2003, p. 5). And second, students become competent writers themselves, in many cases.

Perhaps, most noteworthy about the program is its nonproprietary instructional practices. 90/90/90 schools do not, according to Reeves, adhere to programs that are popularly touted as successful at one given point in time. All programs and strategies are used according to the needs of the student and the expertise of the teacher. This supposed noncommercial way of delivering the program of instruction often frees up the educational leaders and teachers to find and implement any program to advance the 90 percent passing rate.

Indeed, an exciting claim is made that this system is able to achieve such great results for such a poor and underserved population. With poverty figures growing and dropout rates increasing, we need to find solutions and begin meaningful reform for the good of the individual and the good of society. In researching the 90/90/90 schools, we found that none were specifically listed for high academic results. The belief that without any particular service network in place, without attention to healthcare and nutrition, and without family support, 90 percent of students will achieve 90 percent proficiency it too good to be true.

Justin Baeder (2011) examined a list of schools and found results on the WRCT (Wisconsin Reading Comprehension Test) that some, 90 percent of the students did indeed receive a "basic" score. But *basic* is far from proficient. The notion that "data and accountability can help all schools to help all students reach high academic standards was codified in No Child Left Behind. The past decade has seen a nation-wide experiment to determine if Reeves was right. Apparently he wasn't" (n.p.).

Summary

Becoming more intolerant, more insensitive, and more segregated, physically and emotionally, is troubling for the future of our country. Comments are applauded when policy makers and candidates for our leadership in the nation state, "If you don't work, you don't eat." Michelle Bachmann stated that "health care is a privilege," and Senator Jim DeMint condemned the nation's health locally and in the international marketplace. The financial costs to the economy of poor health, lack of education, and higher unemployment are too great to either ignore or to revile.

In this chapter, we have examined the change in direction for civil rights, the resegregation of schools, and an achievement gap that continues to grow in the public school system. All research has pointed to the need for health care beginning prenatally to assure an optimum delivery; early childhood preventative care for healthy growth; and family support for cognitive growth and strength in school. In studies connecting low academic performance (achievement gaps), scientists have found on average, that socioeconomic status predicts a battery of key mental abilities with deficits showing up in kindergarten and continuing through middle school. The stress of poor environmental conditions has been shown to have considerable effects on memory and concentration.

In addition, a study done by researchers at the Institute of Education at the University of London concluded that "there was no link between family structure/instability and a child's' cognitive ability, but persistent poverty had a profound and negative effect on a child's cognitive ability at 5 years of age" (n.p.).

Schools have an opportunity and need to provide programs that are structured and meaningful, but cannot hope to change the early effects on young children who reside in situations that cause malnutrition, stress, poor health care, and education deprivation. Examining schools and their services, one has to consider seriously the holistic approach of the Harlem Children's Promise Academy. Providing early community health care, early childhood education programs, parenting classes, and support, the school has positive results for children and their families.

Important to note that other charter schools serving low-income families have also been successful academically. Comparing the charter schools to the public schools outcomes reinforces the important effects parents have on their children's success. For, all charter schools call for parental knowledge, involvement, and motivation to place their children's names in a lottery system to gain admissions—showing the necessity of family involvement in better schooling that often leads to a better future.

We are not suggesting that conditions such as parental education and income, family structure, parental employment, protection from crime, and child health are not related to students' achievement. Such statistical associations are at the empirical heart of broader, bolder claims. However, evidence, for example, that single parenthood is negatively associated with children's academic achievement is not clear. Rather investment in community services can help to keep families together successfully.

And, we cannot ignore a cascading positive impact on the academic achievement of children in families that are served by marital counseling programs. Per our recitation of findings from studies of Moving to Opportunity, Head Start, and so on, efforts to affect achievement in school through broad interventions outside of school have mixed levels of success.

We thus need to begin educating a total society, where children can become productive, informed participants in adult life—contributing to the democratic process and a better social order. Schools may lead the way, but communities, service agencies, and governments must supply the funds, ideas, and networks for success.

References

Atler, J. (2011). Don't believe critics: Education reform works. *Bloomberg View.* Retrieved from http://www.bloomberg.com/news/2011-06-03/don-t-believe-critics-education-reform-works-jonathan-alter.html.

Aud, S., Hussar, W., Planty, M., Snyder, T., Bianco, K., Fox, M., Frohlich, L., Kemp, J., & Drake, L. (2010). *The condition of education 2010* (NCES 2010–2/28). Washington, DC: National Center for Education Statistics, Institute of Education Sciences, U.S. Department of Education.

Bachman, M. (2011, November 7). Speech as GOP Presidential Hopeful at The Family Research Council.

Baeder, J. (2011, May 11). The 90/90/90 schools myth. *Education Week.*

Brooking (2010).*The Harlem Children's Zone, promise neighborhoods, and the broader, bolder approach to education.* July 20. Retrieved from www.brooking.edu/reports/2010/0720_hcz_whitehurst.aspx.

Brooks, D. (2007) *New York Times* Opinion. Retrieved from www.nytimes.com/2000/05/08/opinion/08brooks.html.

Brown v. Board of Education of Topeka, 347 US 483, 74 S. Ct. 686, 98 L. Ed. 873 (1954).

Dillon, S. (2011, November 5) Merger of Memphis and county school districts revives race and class challenges. *New York Times.*

Diprete, T., Buchman, C., & Shwed, U. (2009). Paper presented at the Russell Sage Foundation. National Center for Educational Statistics May, 2010.

Institute of Education, University of London (2011). *Long-term poverty, but not family instability affects children's cognitive development.* April 21. Retrieved from www.ioe.ac.uk/51936.html

Orfield, G. (2009). *Reviving the goal of an integrated society: A 21st century challenge.* Los Angeles, CA: The Civil Rights Project, UCLA.

———, & Yun, R. (1999). *Resegregation in American schools.* In E. Frankenberg & G. Orfield (Eds.), *Lesson's in integration: Realizing the promise of racial diversity in American schools.* Charlottesville, VA: University of Virginia Press, pp. 1–33.

Parents Involved in Community Schools v. Seattle School District No.1 et al. certiorari to the US court of appeals for the ninth circuit No. 05–908. Argued December 4, 2006—Decided June 28, 2007.

Ravitch, D. (2011, July 7). Reforming the school reformers. *New York Times Magazine.*

Reeves, D. B. (2003). *High performance in high poverty schools: 90/90/90 and beyond.* Retrieved from http://www.sjboces.org/nisl/high%20performances.

Stevens, Justice John Paul. (2007). Response to the 2007 parents involved in *Community Schools v. Seattle School* No. 1, 551 U.S. (2007).

Woodworth, K. R., David, J. L., Guha, R. Wang, H., & Lopez-Torkos, A. (2008). *San Francisco Bay Area KIPP schools: A study of early implementation and achievement.* Menlo Park, CA: Center for Education Policy SRI International.

Whitehurst, R., & Croft M. (2010). *The Harlem children's zone, promise neighborhoods, and the broader, bolder approach to education.* Washington, DC: Brookings Institute Sunday.

12

Intersecting Health, Education, and Well-Being: The Future

Making the World Work for Kids and Society

This book has interconnected the key qualities of life, from childhood into adulthood—relating children's education, health, and economic futures. We know that these elements are closely related, since children from lower-income families are more likely to live in poorer neighborhoods that often have weaker, lower quality schools. Efforts to give families more educational resources—such as public vouchers, tax breaks for groups contributing to education, and access to available charter schools—have helped. But these "privatization" programs are small and limited, compared to the needs of millions of poor children.

Also, we have seen that healthcare in the United States requires real reform, providing more universal, free, and available quality medical services, including regular check-ups and needed treatments, and greater attention to serious medical problems. Universal public education is a possible model, since education is compulsory and is provided with a K-12 education and often beyond—and the government really helps.

Thus, more and better health services, stronger education, and a more active community all contribute to the "common good" and pay back over and over again; for a better income, higher living standards, and greater consumption that spur the economy.

This final chapter pulls all the means together—schools, family, income, and health—to plan for the future. It's a four-front war, as *educationally* we strive to improve schools and availability of good education for children, into adulthood. *Healthcare* has to be universal and of high quality, to treat children, starting with good prenatal care, carrying over into childhood and adulthood. And *economic opportunities*, the most unpredictable area for society, should be expanded and extended, so *families* can earn a decent living and provide for their children (Mare, 1955).

Thus, the quality of life, our physical health, psychological well-being, and the education of parents and their children are closely and complexly related (Longley, 2009). Children need to grow up in positive, healthy environments—consisting of a supportive home life, good health care, and appropriate schooling—that can create connections to self, home, community, and beyond.

This book has sought both to disconnect poor family's income from their children's inadequate education—and thus to reconnect good schooling with improved job opportunities, better careers, higher income, and a better life and education for the next generation. The toughest reconnection, perhaps, is finding a better medical system for all citizens, regardless of income, including good practices, diagnosis, and treatment of medical problems—early in life.

The time is right, as we are over the cusp in new technologies and businesses, if only young people were prepared to take advantage of the new world. Old jobs are going to disappear, it seems, and new forms of work and occupations are coming on. We just need to make our schools more immediate, high-tech, and interactive, so children can interact, learn, and help each other to develop. Not only is getting a good basic early education critical, but also going on to college and beyond are still important for the future, both for the individual and also the family and the society.

Martin Ford (2009) predicts that the new economy will be drastically changed from today:

> With current and future technological advances, average people whose jobs we are going to simulate away…means the bulk of working people in our population. Let's say at least 50 to 60 percent of the employed population… typical people doing typical jobs. In the United States, about 28 percent of the adult population has a college degree. So many of these average people may have gone to college, but most have not. So our assumption is…at some point down the line, machines or computers will take over a great many of these peoples' jobs. (pp. 9–10)
>
> We did see the growth in yearly earnings for full-time employees increasing between 1975 and 1999, with higher starting and ending points for those with higher education attainment, ranging from a low (no high school diploma) to the highest (advanced degrees), although we do see the leveling out of those advantages with "only" a BA or BS degree. (pp. 9–10)

Our education system, aligned with our economic and industrial change and growth, must adjust. It's a three-step process, as this book has shown.

- *Growth of the Economy*: First we need to ensure that our economy and our nation grow and prosper. Why not, for example, expand our relations with nations such as China and India, as we did with Germany and Japan, in manufacturing and marketing. What would American roads and highways look like today without the BMW, VW, Mercedes Benz, Toyota, Nissan, and Honda? And now it's Hyundai and Kia from South Korea taking the country by storm.

These products are often assembled, tested, and sold in the United States. What will be the next set of products, in the future, from China, India, and the European Union? And how will these new services and products increase employment and technology for the next generation of workers and business leaders in the United States too?

- *New Education for All*: Second, education must become more adaptable, universal, and applicable to the new era and new careers. We know that education starts as basic and universal (e.g., reading, writing, calculations, sciences, history, and foreign languages), using virtual textbooks and computer systems to make knowledge, data, and methods available for all—and instantly. In "Reimagining the Textbook," using the Kindle as a concept, Miles and Cooper (2009, 2010) explained:

> The word "kindle" usually refers to fire, using "kindling," or small pieces of wood, to build a flame. But in today's high-tech marketplace, an electronic reading device called Kindle—marketed by the online bookseller Amazon.com,—has started another kind of fire, igniting competitive forces in a movement to deliver books and other written materials in fast, inexpensive ways that fit more easily into the computer age. (p. 11)

Rather than students lugging around pounds of old, out-of-date textbooks, these new electronic devices could provide "books", data, and research for all students, at lower costs than the old textbooks. Every child should have ready electronic access also to data, learning, and the world.

- *Health Care for Everyone*: Third, as this book has discussed, the medical world should learn about "socialized medicine" from the education world of public schooling—where federal, state, and local funding would become universally available for everyone's better diagnosis, treatment, and healthcare from before birth throughout life. For, according to the American Academy of Pediatrics (2005), "Experiences influence every child's development and learning, and these experiences can be positive or negative, with long term consequences for the child and society" (p. 188).

Thus, access to quality health services, treatment for chronic medical conditions, and availability of vaccines administered to children will help to remove a first blockage to education—poor health. For as students' attendance rates increase based on better health treatment, the children's attention span will be enhanced and learning will be improved by being healthy and feeling well.

The effects of long-term medical care in schools and health clinics can result in improved physical well-being and socioeconomic opportunities, thus improving the overall environment for children who have been largely ignored and invisible. Positive community attitudes and knowledge of a better life are made possible and can result in better health, stronger connections to the school, the neighborhood, and society, and a better life and career. What are the steps?

Step 1: Surviving into School

The United States has the second highest death rate for children among the nations in the modern world—with only Latvia being worse. As Dr. Bert Green (2011) reports for CNN Health:

> An estimated 2 million babies die within their first 24 hours each year worldwide, and the United States has the second worst newborn mortality rate in the developed world, according to a news report. American babies are three times more likely to die in their first month as children born in Japan, and newborn mortality is 2.5 times higher in the United States than in Finland, Iceland or Norway, Save the Children researchers found. (p. 1)

These statistics are upsetting, again challenging us to provide better care for pregnant mothers, such as improved diet and reduced drug use, particularly for minorities and disadvantaged groups. For, as we've shown in this book, the connections are there. Charles MacCormack, the retiring president and CEO of Save the Children, explained in the "report card", how children's lives and survival are based on the direct line between the status of mothers and the status of their children" (www.savethechildren.org/site).

Step 2: Getting into a Good School

The next steps, in the ladder to a good life, are finding and obtaining a quality education, at the primary, secondary, and higher education levels. We have shown the process, involving resources, location, and access to good schools. These efforts are sometimes related to location, good housing, and an informed active community.

• **Finding High-Quality Schools.** Real estate agents involved in home sales can often relate statistics on local school performance for their clients who are looking to moving into specific neighborhoods. For those parents who are relocating and have the resources, they can take these steps: traveling to a new neighborhood, touring schools, speaking to current residents, and exploring other important ways of increasing their options. But even those parents who have fewer resources—using information from state, city, and local statistics—may have a reduced likelihood of finding a good school in their neighborhood. And standard test scores are only one indicator.

Parents can also look at class size, teacher education, extracurricular activities, graduation rates, and even after-school care as qualities that identify a good school for them. For those who are interested in property values and resale opportunities, good schools are attractions—and positive selling points for homes and other real estate.

• **Parents Taking a Stand.** A good example of families stepping up and taking charge is the "Parent Trigger" program in California, where mothers and fathers can assess their children's education and take action if their schools are weak. These parents in about 35 schools are organizing petition drives, fighting the system and the unions that hardly want to see their ailing schools shut down.

As the Heartland Institute explained, "Despite the challenges and setbacks in California, the Parent Trigger concept has the potential to improve student performance by giving parents a powerful role in transforming schools where students have struggled despite past interventions by state and federal governments" (Walberg, 2011, p. 11). Created by the Los Angeles Parents Union and passed by one vote in the California Senate, the Parent Trigger program was enacted into law by the California legislature and has the potential to improve schools by empowering vitally interested parents.

As Joseph Bast et al. (2010) found:

> The Parent Trigger idea is also sufficiently malleable to accommodate different political realities in cities and states across the country. In California and in proposed legislation in Connecticut, regulations would empower school districts to veto efforts by parents, and two of the four options seem tailored to the needs of bureaucracies more than children. More reform-minded states such as Indiana, Michigan, and Minnesota might choose to reject those regulations and replace the weakest reform options with something much stronger, such as vouchers. (p. 3)

The Parent Trigger has the potential to turbo-charge the transformation of education in every state by bringing grassroots "regime change" to public education.

• **Considering Private School Options.** For families who can afford tuition in the private school sector, nonpublic education choice is an another option. Parents have alternatives to moving into good neighborhood public schools, using regional private religious, or nonsectarian institutions, based on their or their child's interests. According to a 2009 report by Maria Glod, public school enrollments numbered just under 50 million, while private schooling attendance was reported then at 3.5 million.

Step 3: Exploring Less Expensive Private-Catholic Schools

Since the immigration of Catholics from Ireland, Italy, and Eastern Europe to the United States in the nineteenth century, growing during the Irish Potato Famine in 1850–1855, American Catholic schools have served their families' needs, often at little or no cost (the parish paid for Catholic schools). However, as the Irish and Italians have assimilated and become among the richest ethnic groups in America—and often moved to the suburbs—the inner-city Catholic schools in Washington, DC, New York City, Chicago, and other cities have struggled to stay open—and have began closing at an alarming rate (Cattaro and Cooper, 2007).

Enrollment in Catholic schools peaked in 1965 at 5.66 million and has since declined nationally to 2.2 million students attending. The number of schools likewise dropped, from 14,456 in 1965 to 7,352 schools in 2011. And the decline continues, depriving poor, inner-city parents of the option to select a lower-cost private school, in many cases.

Taking up the slack in some cities, charter schools offer a "privatized" school, often run by private groups and associations, paid for by public funds. But even these charter schools cannot absorb the large number of students who want and need them. Thus, in Milwaukee and Cleveland, for example, charter schools have had to select students using a lottery system, since they cannot enroll the growing number of poorer children who are seeking access.

And poor children who gain admission, based on a random draw, have few chances of being chosen. Thousands of families applied for their children's admission; and the "lottery system" could select only about 10 percent of the applicants—simply because of not having enough classroom space.

Whatever the methods of choice and opportunity in use, we can see the United States is expanding choice through vouchers and charter schools to give lower-income parents a choice of schools and to "break the monopoly" of the public school system by helping to pay tuition to private schools. This trend to offer choice, at public expense, is growing; and we need to see just how well graduates of charter schools do in getting their high school diplomas, and going and graduating from college in the future.

• *School Restructuring:* Public schooling has worked to reform its mission to get more students ready for college, regardless of pre-existing conditions or experiences. Looking toward the future and increasing technological advances, the United States is focused on expanding pre-college academics for all students. Vocational training, with less "academic" courses, has all but been eliminated from options for students less interested or ready for post-secondary education.

We find, in fact, according to U.S. Bureau of Labor Statistics (2010), that jobs and careers are in demand may not always require a college degree: e.g., careers in health related fields, computer support specialists, hair dressing and cosmetology and auto service, real estate agents, technicians and other mechanics.

Step 4: Getting a Good Job

College graduates at the bachelor's levels are now equivalent to what a high school diploma would gain as far as lifetime earnings and wage possibilities are concerned. Many advanced degrees—either professional training, masters, or higher—are now required to obtain more complex skills and higher potential earning power.

And it is true that some professions, no matter their graduate degree designations, have higher earning potential than others. An educator, even with a PhD, might well earn much less than an engineer or an architect— or even a nondegreed electrician or plumber. Thus, Day and Newburger (2002) found that while school reform is geared to college preparation, the service and technological skills in the population are still in demand.

The study further reported:

In 1975, full-time, year-round workers with a bachelor's degree had 1.5 times the annual earnings of workers with only a high school diploma. By 1999, this ratio had risen to 1.8. Workers with an advanced degree, who earned 1.8 times the earnings of high school graduates in 1975, averaged 2.6 times the earnings of workers with a high school diploma in 1999. (Day and Newburger, 2002, p. 2)

A recent survey of school guidance counselors, conducted by College Board's Advocacy and Policy Center by Catherin Gewertz (2011) provides a broad perspective on middle- and high-school students' education and preparation for college:

> Nine in ten counselors, for instance, said that two objectives should top their schools' priority lists: ensuring that all students have access to high-quality education and that they graduate well equipped for college and careers. But fewer than four in 10 said their schools actually operated as if those goals were central to their mission. (Gewertz, 2011, p. 1)

And this "disconnect" between school and employment was even greater in poor, low-income schools: "Only 19 percent of counselors in high-poverty schools said that college and career readiness was part of their schools' day-to-day mission, compared with 30 percent of counselors overall" (Gewertz, 2011, p. 1).

Americans Staying in School Longer

Going and staying in school have changed, as the demand for and benefits of more education have grown. We see children starting their education earlier, at ages 3 or 4, as preschools and prekindergartens have expanded—in part because women are going back to school and to work themselves. And education continues throughout life, with adults expanding their knowledge base and even changing fields.

For even though a college Liberal Arts degree is good preparation, it may not lead directly to a well-paying job. So even college graduates are turning to training and professional development, to obtain "saleable skills" in business, law, medicine, education, engineering, and of course "high tech" fields.

We thus see important changes in the workforce, based on getting a better and more extended education, and a changing economy. While Americans are on average staying in school longer, they are still struggling to find jobs when they graduate, even women who often delayed employment to raise a family.

Greenhouse (2009) reported, "Many of these women are sending out job applications for the first time in years because their husbands were laid off, fear being laid off or had their salaries cut or because their family's investments plunged in value... According to some economists, these women, once part of a privileged minority that could afford not to work, are now collateral damage of the recession—not forced out of work, but back into it." (p. 81).

And like men, women earned more and did better with more and higher education, with the younger women now surpassing the men in graduation from both high school and college and getting better-paying jobs. So in a way, women are illustrating the power of education in their earning power and job opportunities. Thus, schools must attend to the needs of men, and particularly men of color and Latinos, if these groups are to thrive and be able to raise a family to higher levels. It's all interconnected (Levin, et al. 2007).

More and Better Education—*Higher Income*

The more and better an education that children receive, the greater potential they have for higher earnings and a healthier and better life. And although data from the US Bureau of Labor Statistics show that average median earnings increase as levels of education go up, little mention is made about benefits to those in vocational and service careers. Good vocational training is also an important form of education that should be offered and compared to proficiencies outside of the academic scale. Education is essential for all potential workers in the United States, whether it be postsecondary in college, vocational, or service oriented, or on-the-job training.

What would the earnings statistics look like if we compared degrees in academia, or institutions with results from a vocational careers? As previously illustrated, people who finished high school earned almost $175 more each week compared with those who dropped out of high school. If more choice in career were offered, would we prevent higher dropouts and see a more accurate comparison of wage earnings? Can we, as a society, afford not to fund the programs and training necessary to create a workforce that can sustain our economy, by contributing to their and their children's health, education, and well-being?

Conclusion

Extensive research shows both the *inequalities* in school funding (based on local property value, state and local policies) and the effects of *underfunding* on school quality and student outcomes. We need to drive our dollars right down to the classroom, to pay for direct learning services and materials, and help to end the overspending on administration and management. Recent cuts in state spending in New York once again underscored the importance of fairness (equity) in funding, so states can live up to their responsibilities, and do well in comparison to other high-performing nations by driving dollars to teachers and their classrooms.

For example, Billy Easton (2012) identified the problem in an editorial in the *New York Times*:

> Around the world, countries with the top-performing schools, like Finland, Singapore and Canada, all emphasize equity in school financing to provide added resources for schools in poorer communities. These international leaders also emphasize ensuring that all students have access to a high- quality curriculum and providing all teachers with support to continuously improve their skills—instead of forcing teachers and schools to compete for artificially limited pools of money. (Easton, May 25, 2012, p. 21)

School resources belong with and for the child. And funds for health and dental care are greatly reduced for families who need them, even when these services are nearby. Our system of medical services needs to be made available and affordable, for all. Perhaps with help from schools that are nearby and familiar organizations, we can better enable our children to be healthy and well.

And local, state, and federal education policies and funding really matter. The greatest education program ever, the G. I. Bill (the Servicemen's Readjustment Act of 1944), was passed to help millions of World War II veterans returning to civilian life.

Amazing results in just 12 years: for by 1956, over 2.2 million soldiers and sailors had attended colleges and universities and another 6.6 million had obtained needed vocational and technical training, which transformed the workforce and the professions (Bound and Turner, 2005). This economic growth in the United States in the 1950s into the 1960s would not likely have occurred without the millions of veterans who got their education and entered the economic world prepared.

We can consider the G. I. Bill as a great political and economic program, particularly when compared to the poor treatment of World War I veterans who suffered in their efforts to return to civilian life, scarred by unemployment, the Great Depression (1929), and a lack of training for life. The G. I. Bill thus continues to serve veterans of Vietnam and current Middle Eastern conflicts, including their families, and society, to a point where one-third of Americans and their dependents have benefited from these programs over the years, in the reauthorizations of veterans laws. (Humes, 2006).

Bound and Turner (2002) further explain that the G. I. Bill has really "democratized" higher education—and brought educational benefits to generations of Americans—as the conditions were right and still important, including (1) large cohorts of adults needing education after military service; (2) funding made available for both higher education and technical training over time; (3) a rising number of adults prepared for jobs and professions; and (4) increased family incomes, greater industrial and commercial growth, and an improved economy. This model has inspired other federal education programs, and should be continued and increased, based on new markets, needed skills, and increased job opportunities in a changing economy.

How much is further and higher education worth in cold hard money (income)? While some college degrees may mean more in lifetime earnings than others, research into service and technician professions also finds that some in these areas often earn far more. Romero (2008) reports in *Times US*, that a master plumber can earn more than $100,000 annually, while a journeyman plumber usually has a salary of at least $46,000.

Thus, while schools are promoting college as a way to earn more in a lifetime than those who do not attend, diversity in curriculum to accommodate all levels of interest, training in physical and technical skills and abilities will likewise strengthen our economy and provide greater employment across groups and class lines.

And as a nation, we need to pay more attention to our schools, their quality, and productivity, as the foundation agency of our future. Recently, Eli Broad was upset by the declining performance of our education system, and the need to pay greater attention to students' performance in American schools, compared to other nations. Broad (2012) wrote, alarmingly:

American students today rank 31st in the world in mathematics and 23rd in science. If the academic rankings of our most precious resource—our young people—reflected the rankings of our Olympic athletes, it would be a source of national embarrassment. The shameful part of the picture— the one I consider the civil rights issue of our time—is the dramatically lower graduation rates for poor and minority students. These students are far less likely to have access to the best teachers. (December 5, 2012, p. 28)

This book has also detailed the steps in decentralizing the budget to the school—thus putting greater authority in the hands of teachers and school leaders; and coordinating services (e.g., intellectual, physical, medical, dental, and psychological) at the school site.

We need to allocate more flexible dollars to schools, for building better skill-building programs, to make and expand major reforms. And equally important, how can we expand and improve access to universal medical care in the United States? With this comes more and better higher and further education, using the successful 60-plus year G. I. Bill perhaps as a good model for now and the future.

Thus, these improvements in education, health, and life should greatly increase the capacity of families and society to interconnect the world of our children—so they can grow up to be, to paraphrase Benjamin Franklin, healthy, wealthy, and wise!

References

American Academy of Pediatrics (2005, January 1). Quality early education and childcare from birth to kindergarten. *Pediatrics, 115*(1), pp. 187–191.

Bast, J., Behrend, B., Boychuk, B., & Oestreich, M. (2010, August 10). The "Parent Trigger" in California: Some lessons from the experience so far. *Heartland Institute Policy* Brief.

Bound, J., & Turner, S. (2002, October). Going to war and going to college: Did World War II and the G. I. Bill increase educational attainment for returning veterans? *Journal of Labor Economics, 20*(4), 784–815.

Broad, E. (2012, May 23). Never let a crisis go to waste. *Education Week Commentary, 31*(32), 28, 24.

Cattaro, G. M., & Cooper, B. S. (2007). Developments in Catholic schools in the USA: Politics, policy, and prophecy. In G. R. Grace & J. O'Keefe (Eds.), *International handbook of Catholic education—Challenges for school systems in the 21st century* (pp. 61–83). London & New York: Springer.

Day, J. C., & Newburger, E. C. (2002, July). The big payoff: Educational attainment and synthetic estimates of lifetime earnings. US Census Bureau, Population Division. *Special Report.*

Easton, B. (May 25, 2012). Albany's unkindest cut of all. *New York Times*, p. 21.

Ford, M. (2009). *The lights in the tunnel: Automation accelerating technology and the economy of the future.* New York and Paris, France: Acculant Publishing.

Gewertz, C. (2011).How much will the common core cost: Education Week. November 19. Retrieved from http://www.edweek.org/ew/

Glod, M. (2009, June 8). Enrollment in U.S. expected to set record. *Washington Post.*

Green, Bert. (Spring, 2011). Why is infant mortality still a US problem? Retrieved from http://article.wn.com/view/2011/11/02/Why_is_infant_mortality_still_a_US_problem/.

Greenhouse, S. (2009, September 9). Recession drives back to the work force. *New York Times*, p. 81.

Heartland Institute (2010). *The parent trigger: A model for transforming education.* Retrieved from http://heartland.org/policy-document/parent-trigger-model-transformong-education.

Humes, E. (2006). *Over here: How the G.I. Bill transformed the American dream.* Boston, MA: Harcourt.

Levin, H. M., Belfield, C., Muennig, P., & Roused, C. (2007). The public returns to public educational investments in African-American males. *Economics of Education Review, 26,* 700–709.

Mare, R. D. (1995). Changes in educational attainment and school enrollment. In Reynolds Farley, (Ed.), *State of the Union: America in the 1990s,* vol. 1: Economic Trends (pp. 155–214). New York: Russell Sage Foundation, 1995.

Miles, M., & Cooper, B.S. (2009, November 11), "Reimagining the Textbook: The Risks and Reward of Electronic Reading Devices." *Education Week, Commentary,* Vol. 11, pp. 54–55. Reprinted in *California Classroom Science.* January 2010, Vol. 21, Issue 3, p. 1 and 12. (California Science Teachers Association, Sacramento, CA).

Romero, F. (2008). How much do plumbers really make? *Time U.S.* online@www.time.com/time/nation/article/0,8599,1851673,00htm.

Walberg, H. J. (2011). *Achieving more, spending less in schools, districts and states.*

Lincoln, IL: Center on Innovation and Improvement.w

Author Index

Subject Index